A Nutritional Approach to a Revised Model for Medicine

Is Modern Medicine Helping You?

A Nutritional Approach to a Revised Model for Medicine

Is Modern Medicine Helping You?

by

Derrick Lonsdale M.D.

Strategic Book Publishing and Rights Co.

Copyright © 2013 Derrick Lonsdale M.D.. All rights reserved.

No part of this book may be reproduced or transmitted in any form or by any means, graphic, electronic, or mechanical, including photocopying, recording, taping, or by any information storage retrieval system, without the permission, in writing, of the publisher.

Strategic Book Publishing and Rights Co.
12620 FM 1960, Suite A4-507
Houston TX 77065
www.sbpra.com

ISBN: 978-1-61897-092-3

DEDICATION

To my late wife, Adele

The late James P. Frackelton M.D. Partner and friend who taught me much in the practice of Alternative Medicine.

CONTENTS

Preface ix
Introduction xi
Chapter 1: Cultural Decline 1
Chapter 2: A Thumbnail Sketch of the History
  of Medicine 12
Chapter 3: We Have Two Brains 33
Chapter 4: The Fundamental Role of Energy 54
Chapter 5: A Revised Medical Model 68
Chapter 6: How Does the New Model Fit the Practice
  of Medicine? 93
Chapter 7: Opportunist Organisms 114
Chapter 8: Clinical Examples 133

I have a rich experience of patients who have been helped by the art of nutritional therapy. The body is a self-healing "machine" and we can see natural healing aided by these relatively simple methods. Some of the clinical examples, told in every day language, are illustrative. I never use the word "cure," and I tell my patients that I do not "treat disease." I treat the person who has the disease with nutrients in an effort to boost the natural defensive and self-healing mechanisms that we all possess.

PREFACE

Alternative Medicine

The theme of the book is that high calorie malnutrition is a modern scourge that can be compared to the then unknown danger of lead poisoning experienced by the Roman civilization. Historical evidence has been collected and published to claim that the ancient Roman civilization was destroyed at least partly because of this factor. From many years of observation and clinical practice, I have become aware of how high calorie malnutrition affects our ability to adapt to our environment. It produces subtle changes in the biochemical mechanisms that govern our emotional and physical adaptive responses. Like the Romans, we are blithely unaware that the essentially hedonistic attraction to sweet tasting foods and beverages undermine these functions. It makes us react to environmental stresses in an abnormal way, thus making us appear to be more primitive in our behavior. I, like other physicians who have changed to the field of alternative medicine, have very good evidence that the present medical model is wrong. The main error is the divorce of the brain from the body and a refusal to recognize the teaching of Hippocrates who said, "Let food be your medicine and medicine be your food." Getting patients to understand the concept that the brain and body work together is extremely difficult and time consuming. Even after spending a long time with an individual patient, I find that the concept is barely understood and much is quickly forgotten. In this book, I try to give the details in every-day language so that people can use the model to help themselves. By pointing out the fact that the limbic system of the brain is a computer, it is possible to fit every alternative medical technique into the picture and provide an explanation for why each of them works. It is not a book that tells the reader exactly what to do, but gives choices and an explanation of how each method can be expected to work within this model.

High calorie malnutrition is an extremely widespread scourge that is affecting literally millions of Americans. The associated changes in behavior have consequently become so common that they are regarded as being normal. Like the Romans, our total unawareness makes us blind to these effects. Anyone who tries to point them out is a "whistle blower" and history recognizes the difficulty of such an endeavor. In an attempt to compare this with the fate of the ancient Romans the first chapter goes into some of the history of their lead poisoning.

The essential idea expressed is that most, if not all, disease is the result of loss of cellular energy from poor diet in much the same way that a car engine loses power if its fuel is different from that which fits its design.

Over time, the erosion in function begins to decline and begins in the brain, the organ most demanding of oxidative metabolism and energy consumption. High calorie malnutrition can be compared with a choked engine in a car, resulting in poor engine performance, and unburned hydrocarbons being discharged from the exhaust.

INTRODUCTION

Chapter 1 reveals the seeds of cultural decline although there were a number of factors in the decline and fall of the Roman Empire, there is a good case for lead poisoning as an important cause. This is compared with the state of "high calorie malnutrition" of today, which may be a similar long term threat to our present civilization. Although lead poisoning was recognized by a few individuals, they were ignored. The fall of the Roman civilization serves as a useful template upon which the mechanisms of inevitable decline can be discussed. Winston Churchill is an excellent example of a modern "whistle blower." The vast majority of people within any culture have no idea that it is occurring until it goes into decline.

Chapter 2 provides a thumbnail sketch of the history of medicine. The ancient Chinese civilization gave us *yin and yang* as the center of the universe. This is examined for its potential meaning in relation to functions of the body and maintenance of health. Discussion centers on the profound nature of this concept as it applies to "balance" and what that means in our adaptive mechanisms of survival. A brief consideration is given to Hippocrates and the fact that his teaching has been ignored, in spite of his fame. Passing over the medieval period, where surprisingly little progress was made, the origins of the present medical model are discussed. The discovery of microorganisms and the history of our attempts to destroy them as a treatment for the diseases that they cause became the spearhead of research. The idea of "killing the enemy" as the major cause of virtually any disease became the paradigm. Even our techniques for immunization are aimed at boosting the defenses against a specific attacking agent, rather than attempting to increase the efficiency of the immune defenses as a whole through proper nutrition and lifestyle. This "aggressive" model is compared with the paradigm shift in thinking which is spawning the new era of *Alternative Medicine*.

This "new" model accepts the powerful relations of the body and mind in electrochemical terms rather than dismissing "psychosomatic" as an explanation for a patient's "subconscious" self deception. Present attempts at preventive medicine are incomplete and the power of good nutrition has been almost totally ignored in mainstream medicine, although that is beginning to change. An overview of this history is important in understanding the way in which modern medicine has evolved, what is wrong with a large part of the model that it uses, and why extensive revision is necessary. A new model is proposed to explain the loss of health which constitutes disease.

Chapter 3 shows that the brain contains a computer and spells out the most important part of the Universal Model for explaining both health and disease. It depends upon our understanding of the limbic system brain as a computer and its constant dialogue with the more sophisticated cognitive or conscious brain. This communication depends upon a chemical "language" by which the computer communicates with the body that it controls and the cognitive brain that acts as an "advisor." An acceptance of some form of evolution, and a realization that all animal brains have been built on the same basic plan, is necessary.

Chapter 4 describes the role of energy metabolism that can be used to explain the present pandemic of "emotional disease" within a biological framework and shows how the breakdown of the dialogue introduces an idea to explain the phenomenon of "madness, murder and mayhem." The limbic system is the

A Nutritional Approach to a Revised Model for Medicine

primitive individual within us all. It controls and presides over all our "animal" functions. Maturation from infancy, through childhood to adult status becomes much easier to understand and we can begin to see why and how development takes place in each one of us and how understanding energy metabolism is so vital.

Chapter 5 discusses how the present classification of disease is erroneous and describes a proposed revision for a medical model. The mechanisms of many different disease conditions can be explained within the proposed model by correlation with defective energy metabolism in the limbic system. It hinges upon the orchestration of all physical and emotional reactions by the computer. Thus, a whole host of conditions that are presently seen as "physical" can be seen in relation to the "mental" state. We can also begin to see why the present era of medical specialization can easily confuse the real issue. This chapter reasons that disease is manifested by loss of efficiency in energy metabolism, affecting our ability to adapt appropriately to environmental change. The biochemist who can ascertain and define the "biochemical lesion" is the health specialist of the immediate future. This chapter places great emphasis on the fact that it is the de-energized computer that is responsible for what is traditionally thought of as psychosomatic disease. Hence, the pandemic of attention deficit, hyperactivity and other similar diagnostic clichés are caused by high calorie malnutrition in literally millions of our children. Following the mainstream traditional model, these children are unfortunately treated with drugs such as Ritalin and it is a reflection of its use to note that the country actually ran out of this drug a few years ago, sending many parents into a state of panic. Some physicians are not aware of the extent of the problem and, in general, our contemporary society has, until recently, accepted that our nutritional standards are acceptable. We should now be aware that the old adage that "we are what we eat" must be replaced by "we behave according to what we eat." There is now some evidence from animal studies that obesity can be connected with inflammatory disease by stimulating a genetically determined mechanism in the hypothalamus (part of the brain). This mechanism remains inactive until a high calorie diet is provided when its activity induces either obesity, inflammation, or both together.

In chapter 6 it becomes relatively easy to see why and how acupuncture, homeopathy, mind/body disciplines, and nutrition fit into the model. They cannot work without consideration being given to the ever-present dialogue between the "two brains" and the body. Some discussion of the validity of energy medicine techniques is provided within this model. It can be seen how medicine inevitably fits into the latest research in physics and mathematics and must, ultimately, become part of the modern search for the Universal Theory of Matter that eluded Einstein. The presently accepted medical model is a "Newtonian" one, since it deals with structural changes in body organs: hence the term "organic disease," considered generally to be the only cause of "real" disease. The model proposed here is "Einsteinian," dealing with the synthesis, storage and utilization of cellular energy.

In the conventional model, functional changes in the relations between the brain and the body are considered to be "psychosomatic" and treatable by "talk therapy," the basis of psychiatry, or the use of drugs. The "new" model is based upon biochemistry and electricity as they affect cellular metabolism and the exchange of information within the body as a whole. Hence, Alternative Medicine techniques involve the use of nutrition, prescription of therapeutic nutrients rather than synthetic pharmaceuticals, and all the variety of methods used to improve intercellular communication. The normal equipment of adaptive ability is improved by stimulating and balancing the biochemistry throughout the body. The limbic brain is regarded as the "conductor" of an "orchestra" where the body organs are seen as the "instruments." The "symphony of health" is brought about by the constant communication between the brain and the body. The most important need is for an adequate supply of energy for every cell involved in the constant interplay.

In chapter 7 the problem of microorganisms that are known as "opportunist" is discussed. In the present era we are constantly being introduced to "new" microorganisms, resulting in infections that we never heard of before. They are really not new at all and have always been present, "waiting in the wings" for the host to become weakened so that their chance of winning is increased. We have seen how the human body defends itself from its natural microscopic predators. The effectiveness of these organisms in causing disease is a sure sign of our increasingly vulnerable state, rather than an increase in their virulence. Attack by anaerobic (oxygen hating) organisms is a good example of the phenomenon and is well understood. These organisms thrive in tissues deprived of oxygen because they can manufacture their required energy without it: Oxygen kills them. Certain organisms that occur in the human bowel as "friends" can become "enemies" when the normal balance between these organisms is damaged. This balance is another expression of yin and yang. An example is provided by discussion of bacteria that are capable of destroying thiamin (Vitamin B1) and causing disease by depriving the host of this vitamin. A better known example is that of Candida (yeast) which is still not accepted by mainstream medicine as a common problem. An illustration of this is given by describing a relatively rare condition known as mucocutaneous candidiasis. This can be used to illustrate the validity of the proposed disease model.

In chapter 8 some patient problems are outlined to illustrate how the proposed model works in a clinical setting. Some vivid accounts of patients illustrate how and why the author was forced to abandon much of the conventional teaching of the day about the causation and the treatment of disease. In each example, it can be seen that the "new" model indicates that the participation of the brain in all disease mechanisms must be taken into consideration. As the "computer" reacts to input, the messages that are automatically distributed represent both "mental" and "physical" adaptation. This continues twenty-four hours a day, whether we are conscious or not, as in sleep. As outlined in a previous chapter, the computer is really a conductor of an orchestra. The instruments are the organs within the body and the adaptive mechanisms that follow represent the "symphony" of health. Automatic reflexes, initiated in the brain computer, govern much more of our behavior than we are consciously aware. If these reflexes are released too easily, without the "advice and consent" of the cognitive brain, the behavior may become more primitive because the primitive nature of man resides in these reflexes. Sexual drive and hunger for food are examples of the most powerful forces that govern our survival reflexes. If they are initiated too easily because of lack of "self control" we become more like cavemen who did not have the restraints of civilization. The mechanism of self control depends upon an adequate dialogue between the two brains described in the foregoing chapters. Finally, I wish to emphasize that these mechanisms are dependent upon normal chemistry in the brain cells.

AIMS AND SCOPE

Why was this book written?

The book is written because of my professional experiences. I was a pediatrician at Cleveland Clinic in Cleveland, Ohio, for 20 years. This is a famous clinic known worldwide. My specialty was dealing with inborn errors of metabolism, conditions that depend completely on a knowledge of biochemistry. Preventive nutrition is the only possible treatment. I was also a consultant in all pediatric conditions and I became aware that large numbers of children were becoming "emotionally" disturbed, not because of bad parenting but because of "junk" food diets that have become the accepted norm in the U.S. Several important cases of both physical and emotional illnesses turned out to be treated successfully by my rapidly expanding knowledge of vitamin therapy and its role in running the basic machinery of the body and brain (1-3).

1. Lonsdale, D; Shamberger, R J. Red cell transketolase as an indicator of nutritional deficiency. Am J Clin Nutr 1980;33:205-211
2. Lonsdale, D. A Nutritionist's Guide to the Clinical Use of Vitamin B1 Tacoma WA Life Sciences Press; 1987
3. Lonsdale, D. Why I Left Orthodox Medicine: Healing for the 21st Century Charlottesville VA, Hampton Roads Publishing Company, Inc. 1994.

Why is the book needed?

It is needed because it contains a very important message. We behave according to what we eat. The ingestion of high calorie, artificial foods and beverages, particularly those that are being consumed as "drugs" in the form of "sweets," causes inefficient metabolism, particularly in the brain because of its high metabolic rate. Thus, this form of marginal malnutrition results in increasing reflex activity in the lower brain, the part of the brain that controls our instinctive and primitive drives, while weakening the suppressive and inhibitory mechanisms of the conscious, higher brain. It is roughly the same effect as produced by alcohol. This is especially true for children whose metabolism is extremely rapid. Nutrients have to supply the needs for growth and development and this form of malnutrition is a major cause of the epidemic of attention deficit and many similar syndromes that have affected millions of children in various degrees of brain dysfunction.

My long experience of treating sick people with nutrients is similar to the experience of other physicians who have written books about vitamin and mineral therapy. My book, however, attempts to explain the mechanism and how and why this has become a national scourge that threatens the long-term survival of the culture.

What will it cover?

It will cover lead poisoning as an important causative factor in the ultimate destruction of the ancient Roman civilization, using it as an example and comparing its insidious nature with the results obtained from the modern era involving high calorie malnutrition. It will then emphasize the influence of the ancient Chinese civilization in giving us the philosophy of yin and yang and how that introduces the concept of balancing factors in body/brain function. Going on from there it will cover the process by which the field of nutrient based medical treatment has developed because of a growing realization of what is wrong with the present medical model.

How much breadth and depth is there and what is special about the style and approach?

This is an approach that is different from the many books that deal with a "do-it-yourself" description of the use of various nutrients that can be purchased from health food stores. It describes why these are beneficial and the mechanisms involved in helping the healing process. Emphasis is placed upon the need for a new medical model to explain both health and disease

What is special about the author?

I have 64 years of practicing medicine. I was educated in England and graduated from London University with the degree, M.B. B.S. in 1948. After graduation, I became a family doctor in Britain and emigrated to the U.S. in 1960 when I became a pediatric, Board Certified specialist at Cleveland Clinic until 1982. I then went into private practice, specializing in nutrient-based treatment derived from my clinical research experiences.

For some years I was an advisor to the Board of Trustees of the American College for Advancement in Medicine (ACAM) and edited its medical journal, *Clinical Practice in Alternative Medicine*, published by Innovision Communications Inc. The combination of clinical practice and research has given me a unique knowledge about the reasons for how and why alternative medical practice needs to be integrated into mainstream medicine. It is certainly a rapidly growing trend in America.

CHAPTER 1

THE SEEDS OF CULTURAL DECLINE

Each species in the animal kingdom has evolved by adapting to its environment. We consider ourselves to be the most sophisticated species and our evolutionary adaptation has been inevitably linked to our ability to use tools and to think. It has led to a great deal of artificiality in protecting us from the harsh reality of existence. Consequently our history has involved many structured societies. Each has risen to a zenith of achievement and then declined. Hancock made a convincing case that a very advanced culture was in existence thousands of years ago and was destroyed by a cataclysmic event of gargantuan proportions (Hancock, G. *Finger-prints of the Gods,* New York, Crown Publishers, Inc). He suggests that "it had to begin all over again and that the renewal was guided by a few survivors of the destructive natural event."

Cultures have appeared and disappeared like weather systems. Historians, archeologists, and anthropologists are sometimes at a loss to explain why an organized society disappeared. The decline which we see in our own civilization is fairly obvious. Within a given culture, how many members of it possess the ability to perceive the mechanism of its inevitable decline? Even if there are such individuals, do they really have any effect on the outcome?

The civilization of ancient Rome has often been compared with the present day and this chapter seeks to use one aspect of their decline in comparing it with one aspect of our own.

Hedonism was, of course, a well known part of the decline, but there is circumstantial evidence that at least part of the decay within the Roman Empire was related to chronic lead poisoning. An article was published in the *Journal of Occupational Medicine*, entitled "Lead poisoning and the Fall of Rome" by S.C Gilfillan. There was a gradual disappearance of science after the second century and a retreat from almost all that had spelled "the glory that was Greece and the grandeur that was Rome." He offered a completely new explanation for the Roman decay, derived from studies of toxicology, vital statistics, archeology, bones, recipes, and lead-lined pots from brewing poisons "considered delicious by the ancient well-to-do because of their sweet taste induced by the presence of lead." Although recognizing many other factors, lead poisoning was an important component in the decline.

The symptoms of lead poisoning, still a potent industrial disease, are unfamiliar to most. Continued daily intake in an amount greater than 1 mg may be dangerous, only 1/28,300 of an ounce. Chronic constipation and colic, conspicuous symptoms, were recorded by the Romans. Other symptoms include headache, insomnia, blindness, and mental disturbances extending to insanity. "Crazy as a painter" was a common phrase not long ago when lead based paint was used. Gilfillan emphasized loss of fertility in men and women who suffered sterility, miscarriage, stillbirth, or premature labor. Children born to such women are apt to die shortly after birth. Children are particularly susceptible, the result being permanent physical or mental damage. Lead poisoning is still a widespread problem in American children. Mercury has a similar action in damaging brain metabolism.

Well-to-do Romans had lead paints and the favorite color of their rich walls was Pompeian red, produced by minium, a salt of either lead or mercury, the latter also being a common poison today. Perhaps the major part of Gilfillan's argument was derived from many studies that lead poisoning of the wives and mistresses of upper-class Romans occurred chiefly through their diet, after the introduction of Greek cooking around 150 B.C. and the relaxation of the rule against wives drinking wine. The most significant sources of lead were wine, grape syrup, and preserved fruit. The Roman free poor and slaves had much less lead in their diet, because these dietary pleasures did not exist for them to such a degree. Gilfillan noted that it was the rich Romans who were made childless, leaving the inheritance of the culture to the less capable who were unable to pick up the responsibilities of government. In comparison, it is now known that Vitamin B1 deficiency, induced by an excess of sugar, can cause a decrease in the sperm count. Infertility is common today.

Why were the ancient rich so reckless as to drink lead compounds daily? Nicander, in the second century B.C. had described poisoning in lead workers and their physicians knew about it, but the only reference to its occurrence in foodstuffs was made by Vitruvius in a treatise written in the first century. It was certainly not a well known danger, in spite of the fact that 2,100,000 tons of lead were produced in 300 years in the silver mines of Laurion, the fountain of prosperity in Athens. In these mines, 300 ounces of lead were produced for every ounce of silver. To illustrate its almost profligate usage, a salvaged Greek wine ship of about 150 B.C. had 200 tons of cast lead sheathing tacked onto it.

Lead was cheap, easy to smelt and they put it into their wine in as many as fourteen different ways. It poisoned the microorganisms that cause fermentation and souring, but they did not know that they were sterilizing themselves. Of hedonistic significance, lead gives a slightly sweetish taste, thus contributing to the drunken orgies that became so common.

A picture in an old issue of the *National Geographic* magazine showed an ancient smelter in action. The smoke contained a large amount of lead. In Greenland's ice, French geologists have found lead levels that were derived from fires in ancient Europe between 500 B.C and 300 A.D. enough lead was precipitated in the Arctic snow to equal fifteen percent of the lead deposited there by burning leaded gasoline from 1930 to1990. In their heyday, the smelters produced 90,000 tons of lead ingots a year. John P. Oleson of the University of Victoria agreed that Romans ingested enormous quantities of lead in their food and drink. They flavored food with boiled-down grape juice that derived much of its sweetness from leaden cooking pots.

Few contemporary individuals knew what was happening, or if they did, they were helpless to do anything about it. If there was someone who was sufficiently knowledgeable, could see the impending disaster, and had the strength and the courage to become a "whistle-blower," what would have been his fate? It is probable that such a person would have had no attention paid to him. Only history can look back and see what happened and why. We seem to be collectively powerless to control our destiny.

Oswald Spengler wrote, "The decline of the West, which at first sight may appear like the corresponding decline of the Classical Culture, we now perceive to be a philosophical problem that, when comprehended in all its gravity includes within itself every great question of Being." He noted that Napoleon has hardly ever been discussed without a side-glance at Caesar and Alexander. Mankind is rightly reckoned as one of the organisms of the earth's surface, its physical structure, its natural functions, all belong to a more comprehensive unity. He added that there is no analogous case of one culture making a passionate cult of the memory of another. He also said that it "remains now to sketch the last stages of western science. The gently sloping route of decline in our own age is clearly visible. Through money, democracy becomes its own destroyer; after money has destroyed intellect. In no other civilization has the will-to-power manifested itself in so inexorable a form as this of ours."

Galileo said that nature is written in mathematical language and every culture, every springtime, every rise and fall, has its determined phases which invariably recur with the emphasis of

A Nutritional Approach to a Revised Model for Medicine

a symbol, Every being of any import, from intrinsic necessity, recapitulates the phases of the culture to which it belongs.

Robert L. Heilbroner, in *An Inquiry into the Human Prospect* in 1974 provided some bleak statistics. World population at that time was about 3.6 billion, of which 1.1 billion resided in North America, Europe, Japan, Oceania, and the former Soviet Union. This population was expected to become stable within two generations, but will still increase by thirty to forty percent. On the other hand, Southeast Asia will double in thirty years, Africa in twenty-seven years, Latin America in twenty-four years and the underdeveloped nations will eventually have to support forty billion. Even in 1967 the report of the President's Science Advisory Panel on World Food Supply stated that malnutrition in the underdeveloped nations was estimated to affect sixty percent of the population. Increases in rural population, leading to redundant manpower and unemployment, gives rise to a flood of desperate people into the cesspools of the cities.

Heilbroner noted that "while men can generally acquiesce in, even relish, the destruction of their living contemporaries, when they can regard with indifference or irritation the fate of those who live in slums, rot in prison, or starve in lands that have no meaning only insofar as they are vacation resorts, why should they be expected to take the painful actions needed to prevent the destruction of future generations whose faces they will never live to see." He also said that "contemporary, industrial man, his appetite for the present whetted by the values of a high-consumption society and his attitude toward the future influenced by the prevailing canons of self-concern, has but a limited motivation to form a collective bond of identity with future generations. It is the absence of such a bond with the future that casts doubt on the ability of nation-states or socioeconomic orders to take now the measures needed to mitigate the problems of the future."

Richard Falk, in *This Endangered Planet*, written in 1971, said that the 1970s would be the politics of despair, the 1980s of desperation, the 1990s of catastrophe and the 21st century the era of annihilation. "The enormous quantities of unusable waste produced for each ton of metal created by the industrial countries are more easily disposed of in a blueprint than in a field." Robert Ayres and Allen Kneese, in *Extended Industrial Revolution and Climate Change* in 1971 noted that the emission of energy was estimated at 1/15,000 of the absorbed solar flux. If the existing rate of growth continued, this energy would reach 100% of the solar flux absorption in 250 years. This would raise the temperature of the earth about fifty degrees C, and render it unsuitable for human habitation. Today, the warnings are multiple and come from many different sources. The application of history is invariably ignored.

In April 1997 the *National Geographic* published a warning. Minnesota schoolchildren, on a field trip in 1995, found that half the frogs that they caught were deformed. Extra legs or missing legs or eyes "have now been found everywhere that frogs are common in our state" according to Robert McKinnell of the University of Minnesota. Nearby states have reported the same phenomenon. Nobody knows the cause but we can surely guess that it is the influence of our reckless outpouring of chemicals.

We have become increasingly deaf to the multiple warnings to which we are repeatedly exposed. The *National Geographic Magazine* publishes such warnings regularly and a recent issue was devoted completely to the evidence for global warming, an effect that is still believed by many to be unrelated to man. Huge increases in world population, disappearance of the rain forest, industrial waste, chemical pollution of the atmosphere, the "greenhouse effect," and many other facets of our failure in stewardship of the earth are common knowledge.

Our Adaptation Depends on Perception

We only "know" that everything in our world exists because of sensory perception. We hear, touch, smell, and see, all functions of the brain. We naturally assume that this represents reality. It is something that has intrigued scientists and philosophers for centuries. One of the best known was the 17th century thinker Descartes, who said, "Because I think, I am."

All animal brains are built on the same basic principle, starting with the lower and oldest part. Built up, layer by layer through evolution, each species has developed a brain that is most suited to its habitat.

As more complexity was added, so have the functions become more diverse. Where in the evolution of species does the phenomenon of conscious awareness begin? We possess consciousness and are capable of appreciating abstract phenomena such as beauty. We understand the basic facts of life and death. We perceive and assess the world in which we live. We do not know how much consciousness exists in other species.

Functionally we really have two brains, the lower and more primitive limbic system and the upper cognitive. Sanity, and the normal behavior that goes with it, is brought about by a dialogue between them. The newborn infant has both parts, but it is only the lower one that is in operation at birth. When the dialogue between the upper and lower brains begins to emerge, as hardwiring continues, there is gradually more sophistication. This is called maturation, summed up by the phrase, "when I was a child I behaved as a child, but when I became a man, I put away childish things."

The child is more primitive, guided much more by the lower brain. Maturation is a process of development leading to brain completion. Sanity represents a full dialogue between the two brains. This allows for all shades of communication between them and enables us to understand that vandalism and otherwise incomprehensible behavior is based upon the loss of "advice and consent" that must constitute an important monitoring function of the upper brain over the lower. I shall return to this theme in more detail later, but I want to introduce this concept early because it is the foundation of the model that I am attempting to describe.

We cannot turn the clock back, even if we wanted to. An experiment was performed in England some years ago when a group of people had the idea that civilization was artificial. They set about living exactly as cave men appeared to have lived, using no modern methods at all. They had to give up. Our adaptive mechanisms have been eroded in the wake of our artificiality. Thus, civilization is our ultimate enemy against our biology.

I always marvel when I see a horse out in a field casually eating grass and manifestly comfortable when the evening is closing down in the winter. We could not do it! We would freeze to death. Then why does the horse not freeze to death? The answer is that there has been no advent of an artificial means to protect the animal from its natural environment. It has evolved within that environment and, if it had not done so, it would have perished as a species.

Agriculture developed as a convenience. It was easier to grow food in the backyard than to look for it in the forest. It has been a search for convenience ever since until the present when we drive a two ton machine to the super-market to buy food that is packaged and processed. It is for our convenience and to save the time that is otherwise required in food gathering and preparation. This goes along with the fact that our society is becoming ever more stressful as it accelerates and attempts to do things faster and faster. There is no time left "to smell the roses," that old cliché. The only question that might be asked in view of this is, "What do we do with the time that is saved?"

We often try to claim that modern medicine is responsible for the increased life span that our statistics reveal. Unfortunately, the statistics do not take into consideration the number of people who are languishing in nursing homes, sometimes for years before they become a death statistic. It was not modern medicine that conquered tuberculosis. It was due to better hygiene, housing, and more adequate nutrition. It should be noted; however, that tuberculosis is returning to the modern scene because of a weakening of our defensive resources, our immunity. It is a foreseeable condition in those afflicted by AIDS, for example.

Our health statistics bear out the facts. Like Gilfillan, who added the factor of lead poisoning to the complexities of the decline in Rome, the mental health of our contemporary society is in jeopardy, and that it is a powerful vector force in our predictable decline. We have about thirty million women affected by the condition known as Premenstrual Syndrome (PMS). Up to about six percent of the population is known to have mitral valve prolapse, a condition which is related to functional changes in the autonomic nervous system. It is reported that five percent of grade school children are receiving Ritalin for behavioral pathology which can usually be easily erased by simply correcting their appalling nutrition. Indeed, those statistics may be an underestimate, for we became aware that the country "ran out" of Ritalin a few years ago and caused panic among the parents whose children are maintained in a state of relative equilibrium by the use of this drug.

Physical disease cannot be separated from brain function. All mental disease is just as physical as body disease is mental. We have, however, concluded that functional changes in the brain affecting the body are "psychosomatic." It is the chemistry of brain that decides what kind of messages go from it to the adaptive functions of the body. Well-balanced and normal chemistry gives rise to normal adaptive changes in the brain and body in response to environmental changes. Abnormal chemistry gives rise to maladaptive mental and body functions. It is the dialogue between the lower brain and the body, and between the lower and upper brain that decides how we adapt to environmental influences. Modern disease was referred to by Hans Selye as "The diseases of adaptation." I believe that an even better term would be, "The diseases of maladaptation.

For every patient whose health is restored by redirecting lifestyle and diet in particular, there are millions who require the same advice. It is an extraordinarily difficult task to get a person to understand what he or she must do in order to restore health which has been declining steadily, sometimes for years. Even if a person has a genuine desire to make the lifestyle changes required, there may not be sufficient acceptance to grasp the extent of the change. It is never easy to persuade a person that health is a personal affair and that we cause our own diseases by the way we approach life. Smoking is the worst habit to eradicate even though the patient invariably knows that it is a major cause of ill health. Who could not know in this day and age? But does it make any difference to the individual? Sometimes, by truly heroic measures and strength of will, smoking cessation is achieved, but it can be worse than alcohol in its addictive action.

The word "doctor" comes from the Latin *doceo*, "I teach." The original meaning of the English word, therefore, was "a teacher." It is only in recent times that the word has been used to indicate a healer. The doctor does not heal anyone. It is the body that heals itself and the doctor must teach the patient how to retrieve his or her own health and that is what the *New Medicine* is all about. We believe that our modern medical technology has created the most advanced "state-of-the-art" ever known. In fact, it is this reasoning that has led to such a vast increase in medical expenses. If technology is good, then more is better. Though I am not denying the benefits that have accrued from this development, it certainly has its "flip" side. Sometimes, unfortunately, we see disease being virtually "invented" by false interpretation of technology. The fear of "missing something" related to the symptoms described by the patient, adds tremendously to the overuse of this technology, thus increasing the costs of medicine profoundly. Technology is a two-edged sword and can be detrimental if it is used without discretion. Our preoccupation with gadgets is a modern whim that goes right through our society. In other ways, technology has damaging effects to our biology.

A Nutritional Approach to a Revised Model for Medicine

The so-called "couch potato"/ television syndrome has three disadvantages. One is that it acts as a substitute for imagination and the thought processes that have enabled us to progress in the evolutional experiment. The second is that it substitutes for the necessary physical exercise that is a vital part of our biologic health. And the third is that it seems to be associated with junk food ingestion. It is often the in-between-meal eating that does the damage, not the three main meals routine. It is very hard indeed to get people to be aware of this and how it works against them. The relationship of diet and health will be made clearer in a later chapter. Suffice it to say that high calorie malnutrition is the modern equivalent of lead poisoning as it affected the Romans.

It is the marketplace that decides the ultimate issue. If the public demands changes in the food industry and in the aggressively dangerous dice-playing of the pharmaceutical industry, we may yet be able to retrieve our collective mental and physical health. But there has to be a major change in our attitude.

CHAPTER 2

A THUMBNAIL SKETCH OF THE HISTORY OF MEDICINE

Early Origins of Theory and Practice

As we explore the functions of our own bodies and become more knowledgeable about the intricacies of its machinery, we become more arrogant in believing that we can either do better than nature or find ways and means of patching its perceived mistakes. Tracing some of the past history of medicine can perhaps give us an idea of how we arrived at the modern drug-based method of treatment. Disease and health have been regarded in various ways ever since man had sufficient brain sophistication to understand the difference. To see how medical thought has developed, we have to start with pre-history. The word holistic comes from the word *holos*, meaning a hill. This came from an ancient language used by people who gathered herbs from the hillside. Thus, the use of herbs has a long lineage and is now beginning to be revived in our modern era. This fact indicates that people are not entirely satisfied with the present methods of "scientific" medicine used today.

We will start with a consideration of medicine as it was practiced by the ancient Chinese. They were extremely observant and developed methods of treatment that were derived from their observations.

Yin and Yang

Later in this book, we will emphasize the importance of "balance" in all the mechanisms of the human body. *Yin* and *Yang* represent a fundamental philosophy that, when applied to body functions, can open the mind to phenomena that become more easily understood. It is therefore valuable to consider how and why such methods were developed and why, for instance, acupuncture is still used some five to ten thousand years later. The Chinese sages who developed acupuncture and pulse diagnosis from careful observation of their patients were true clinical physicians who were not diverted by the technology that we have in modern medicine. We tend to believe that these ancients were less knowledgeable than we are today, since they lived at a time when this technology was not available. I am not, of course, suggesting that we should get rid of the technological advances, but there is a tendency for us to be certain that technology will remove all the "guess-work" from the ultimate goal of ascertaining what is wrong with a sick person. So pervasive is this concept, that modern physicians may perform a CAT scan or other form of imaging before listening to what the patient has to say. We have come to believe that we have developed wonders that make the history of medical science obsolete.

There are several factors that have made the wisdom of ancient China inaccessible to us. The first is the obvious difficulty of the language symbols themselves, and second, that the language speaks in "mind pictures" that must be interpreted. Western medicine evolved without the benefits of this ancient wisdom. We have perceived Chinese medicine as quaint and developed from a state of ignorance rather than knowledge built on observation. I believe that the philosophy of yin and yang represents the most advanced and realistic picture of reality that has ever been devised. To see how it applies to functions of the body and how it makes sense in our modern world, we must take a look at it.

Derrick Lonsdale M.D.

First, the Chinese approach depended upon viewing the body as one whole piece of machinery and that it was well able to carry out its own program of defense. The healing process came from within and was to be assisted in all possible ways. Hence, their preoccupation with nutrition as an appropriate source of body fuel for reaching maximum efficiency. The two prevailing techniques, acupuncture and moxibustion were, and still are, aimed at producing their effect by stimulation. With modern knowledge of how we are constructed, it is probable that they were stimulating that part of the nervous system that deals with our adaptive responses. Such responses depend upon internal messenger systems that receive stimulation from environmental changes.

If something is good for us, more of it may be better, but an excess is bad. That is the very heart of yin and yang. There must always be an optimum state. We do not want to be either hot or cold. To be warm is the point of balance between the two extremes. My acquaintance with ancient Chinese medicine was derived from *A Brief History of the Yellow -Emperor's Classic of Internal Medicine* by Ilza Veith and a *Celestial Lancets* by Jen and Joseph Needham. I quote here liberally from these authors.

Whether Huang Ti, the Yellow Lord, or the Yellow Emperor, was mythical or not is unclear. Geneologies of Chinese dynasties list him as the third of China's first five rulers and ascribe to him the period of 2697-2597 B.C. "The Age of the Five Rulers" is said to have lasted 647 years (2852-2205 BC) and is called the "Legendary Period." The Yellow Emperor is considered to be the author of *Nei Ching Su Wen*, the classic treatise on internal medicine, and supposedly the oldest medical book extant. The development of Chinese medical philosophy even predates this and may have been in existence for centuries before the book was written. What did these philosophers and observers of humanity mean by yin and yang? I found no clear definition, although it became obvious that the two words represented extremes on either side of a median, the equivalent of the "bell-shaped curve" which is so popular with statisticians today. *Tao*, and yin and yang are referred to frequently in the medical canon to which I have referred. Tao is the key to the mysterious intermingling of "Heaven and Earth" and refers to the method of maintaining the harmony between this world and the beyond by shaping earthly conduct to correspond completely with the demands of the "other world." Man, in his utter dependence upon the universe, could do no better than follow a way conceived after that of nature. The only manner in which he could attain the right way, the Tao, was by emulating the course of the universe with complete adjustment to it. We might refer to this in modern terms as a process by which each of us adapts to our environment.

It was inevitable that Tao, in its role as supreme regulator of the universe and the highest code of conduct, should play an important part in early Chinese medical thought, which was so inextricably entwined with philosophical concepts. Numerous references in the *Nei Ching* impress the reader that his health, and with it the highly desirable state of longevity, depended largely upon behavior toward Tao. Longevity itself became, to a certain degree, a token of sainthood since it indicated complete adherence to Tao. References to Tao throughout the *Nei Ching* rarely discuss it alone, but generally in conjunction with the two component parts of the universe, the yin and yang.

Although Yin and Yang have received a vast variety of interpretations, by analyzing the ideographs themselves, the original and basic meaning of the "word picture" characters can be ascertained. This results in "the shady side of a hill" for yin and "the sunny side of a hill" for yang. Other interpretations see them as two banks of a river, one of which is in the shade, the other exposed to the sun. Yin represents the shady, cloudy element while yang stands for the sunny and clear element. If we keep in mind these original meanings, cloudy and sunny, their many connotations become more logical since they mean, in essence, the two extremes on either side of an intermediate state. Other contrasts might be virtue/vice, order/confusion, reward/punishment, joy/sadness, wealth/poverty, or health/ disease. Yang represented the positive and yin the negative side, but must not be interpreted to mean that yin was "bad" and yang was "good." They were always conceived as one entity that, both together, were ever-present. Day changed into night, light to darkness, spring and summer into fall and winter. In other words, all happenings in nature as well as in human life were conditioned by the constantly changing relationship of these two cosmic regulators.

The general application of this duality led to the realization that neither component existed in an absolute state and therefore there was yang within yin, and vice versa. Duality, in other words, was preserved within a single thing. The most concrete example is man himself. As a male, man is yang, but as female belongs to yin. Yet both male and female are contained in both sexes. It was expressed in the *Nei Ching* as "the principle of Yin and Yang is the basis of the entire universe. It is the principle of everything in creation." The book constantly refers to yin and yang in reference to disease and health. Perfect harmony between them meant health and disharmony or undue preponderance of one element brought disease and death. The doctrine of Tao was a way of voluntarily assisting that balance. Hence, "the Yang and the Yin of the universe are called Tao."

This knowledge was considered to be even strong enough to counteract the effect of age. "Those who have the true wisdom remain strong, while those who have no wisdom grow old and feeble." The ideal age for man was one hundred years and this was considered to be due to living in harmony with heaven and earth, yin and yang, and the four seasons. The seasons were regarded merely as the result of the interaction of the two forces that stood for sun and moon, heat and cold, dryness and humidity. This invoked the same mode of life required of any agricultural people at any time and anywhere in the world.

This philosophy says that too little is as bad as too much, but the middle of the road is the correct place to be. That means, of course, that there is something of both extremes that make up a mid-zone for everything. Certainly, modern medical science is showing us clearly that this is true. We need calcium and magnesium in the proper balance and we cannot do without these essential elements, and this theme is reiterated time and time again in our physiology.

Pulse Diagnosis

The chief means of obtaining clinical information from the patient by ancient Chinese physicians was by "pulse diagnosis." This was derived, at least in part from a cultural notion. A physician, invariably male, was unable to have his female patient undressed because of the code of moral conduct that prevailed. This lead to other ways of gaining information about the functions of the body and the pulse was observed patiently and interminably over many years. The patient would sit on a chair with his hands on a table, behind which sat the physician who held both of the patient's wrists with his own fingers on the pulses. Observation told them that there were six different kinds of pulse, three in each wrist. There were four principal pulses described in word-picture terms, but could be translated to indicate superficial, deep, fast and slow.

This may seem to be absurd today but what these wise observers were checking was the continuously changing features of heart speed and strength in regulating the supply of blood to the body. This is an important part of our ability to adapt to the constantly changing state of the environment in which we have to survive throughout our lives. Modern electronic equipment has been able to show that the balance of the autonomic nervous system in regulating heart speed and variability is a vital part of our continuously adapting machinery. The autonomic system works automatically without any conscious control and this is one of the mechanisms that is under stress from our present civilization.

But further than that, in order to find an auspicious moment for his undertaking, the physician had to determine the timing of the examination. It was considered that the best time of day was the early morning when the physician himself was alert. In the words recorded by Ilza Veith, the optimum time was "when the breath of Yin has not yet begun to stir and when the breath of Yang has not yet begun to diffuse, when food and drink have not yet been taken, when the twelve main vessels are not yet abundant and when vigor and energy are not yet exerted."

Because this interpretation seems to us to be strange, we automatically conclude that it was because of observations that were made in a state of ignorance. But consider this in the light of our modern knowledge of physiology. It is becoming ever more clear that the brain rhythm known as Circadian (meaning twenty-four hours) has a fundamental part to play in our physical and mental health. Forget the bizarre wording: it was clear that these people understood that the human body had rhythms that were absolutely vital to health. We now know that this rhythm is an important element in our healthy adaptive mechanisms. These ancient Chinese physicians knew what they were doing when they refused to treat the patient at a certain time of day. Somehow, they recognized that the physical state of the patient was more receptive to treatment, depending upon the time of day.

Acupuncture

Acupuncture is at least 5,000 years old. It relies on the fact that channels of electrical communication exist within the body and that they are a source of constant communication between organs. They rely on a source of energy that is probably electromagnetic in nature and the acupuncture points on the surface of the body represent the "terminals." Acupuncture is now being sought more and more frequently in this modern age because people find that it works. Confidence in the therapeutic value of acupuncture was closely connected with the belief in forces that created the world and whose interaction caused the balance within the universe and within the body. These forces, Yin and Yang, were deemed to balance each other completely but were considered to be in a constant state of flux as in day to night. Within the body, the distribution of the forces was considered to be uneven and the dual power could function only if the flux of yin and yang was uninterrupted. Stagnation on one part, producing a deficiency in another, resulted in disease. Acupuncture is being used today and is very effective for some. It is certainly true that its action is related to the flow of energy that provides necessary communication throughout the body. So much of this philosophy makes sense in the light of our modern knowledge. We now know that the heart and pulse are governed by an extraordinarily complex network of nerves and hormone messengers which create a powerful ability to adapt to rapid changes in both mental and physical circumstances.

The Autonomic Nervous System and High Calorie Malnutrition

The disease known as *beriberi* is an ancient scourge that killed thousands of people throughout the world, including America. It was found to be largely due to a deficiency of Vitamin B1 and is still relevant in parts of the world where rice is the staple. It is the prototype for high calorie malnutrition. Believe it or not, this disease exists today in America in a marginal form and is difficult to spot unless its essential nature is thoroughly understood. It affects the nervous system in certain ways, particularly the "balance" of the autonomic nervous system. Thus, it can be represented by subtle changes in blood pressure and pulse volume that mirror the Chinese observations.

Modern physicians rarely know anything about the classic forms of nutritional disease. They are taught in medical schools in a superficial way only because they are considered to be historical relics. Not knowing the severest forms of these diseases very well, it is difficult, if not impossible, to recognize symptoms caused by mild or marginal malnutrition.

High calorie malnutrition is quite different from starvation and I have likened it to choking an internal combustion engine. It is the consumption of foods that may be tasty and satisfying, but have insufficient accompanying vitamin/mineral components, the path towards the appearance of beriberi if developed to the fullest. For example, many of the children that I have seen with a variety of symptoms, caused by their high calorie malnutrition, have high systolic and low diastolic blood pressures. In fact, the diastolic pressure is sometimes zero, together with an unusually high systolic pressure, a signature of autonomic nervous system change that is most characteristic in *beriberi*. Blood pressure in children is often ignored by pediatricians because hypertension is considered to be an adult condition. There are, however, some interesting subtleties in taking blood pressures in children that can tell us a great deal about how the brain is regulating the complex associations between the heart and the blood vessels. Blood pressure changes of this nature are seen in association with behavioral abnormalities that have become so common in the children of today. These subtle changes disappear with correction of diet and supplementation with vitamins and minerals. It is not surprising that Vitamin B1 is frequently the most important vitamin to be required as a supplement since it is of vital importance in normal metabolism of sugar.

Pulse Pressure

The difference between the systolic and diastolic blood pressure is known as the pulse pressure. For example, in a child with an abnormal blood pressure of 100/0 the pulse pressure is 100. One month later, after correcting the high sugar diet and providing appropriate vitamin/mineral supplementation, the blood pressure of 90/60 is now normal and the pulse pressure 30. The child is reportedly calmer and much less "psychologically" handicapped.

A Nutritional Approach to a Revised Model for Medicine

What this means, of course, is that the communication between the heart, the blood vessels, and the brain computer has been radically changed. It must have been that the sensitive and practiced fingers of the ancient Chinese physicians, feeling the pulse at the wrist, had been able to detect such a change. What they were measuring, although they did not have the scientific knowledge that we have today, was a state of imbalance in the adaptive control systems of the body.

The Chinese observations can be quite relevant in our determination of what is wrong with so many people in today's world. It is clear that the emphasis was preventive. It was said that "those who disobey the laws of Heaven and Earth have a lifetime of calamities, while those who follow the laws remain free from dangerous illness." We are learning today, at least in the field of Complementary Alternative Medicine that this is a fundamental truth. "The ancient sages did not treat those who were already ill; they instructed those who were not ill." As a simpler life gave way to more noxious influences, it became necessary to develop new methods. Minor illnesses became more severe and death from them more common.

The second method of treatment was through diet, founded at that time on "the five elements and the concordances based thereon," although this has no meaning to us today.

I quote again from the book by Ilza Veith. "Smooth movement of breath and blood present the most advantageous conditions for the flow of Yin and Yang. Stagnation can be caused by a plethora of Yang or a deficiency of Yin. Either state can occur independently, or one can be the cause of the other." Both of these failings were indicated by the pulse beats. Later on, we shall be thinking more about the way balance is maintained in our adaptive mechanisms as we understand them today and how this involves the brain/body association.

Cyrano de Bergerac, in his 1659 philosophical voyage to the countries of the Moon and the Sun, discusses the power of the mind with his guide, the Daemon of Socrates. Cyrano says,

"I have known more than twenty miraculous cures of men who were sick unto death!" The Daemon, in his reply, refers to the power of the mind,

"This is why the ablest physicians on your earth advise a patient rather to take an ignorant doctor, whom he esteems to be very knowing, rather than a skilful physician whom he imagines to be ignorant. The most powerful medicines will be too weak if the imagination does not apply them. Are you surprised that the most ancient men of your world lived to so many ages without the least knowledge of being physically sick? Their nature was yet in force, their constitutions were resilient, and that universal balsam had not yet been dissipated by the drugs wherewith your doctors consume you."

Balance applies to the chemistry and physiology of the body. The ancient Chinese described their observations in pictorial language. They were able to perceive the "point of balance" between yin and yang and likened it to "a flock of birds" or "the breeze in the waving millet." It was stressed that "only too easily can one miss the fleeting moment" and acupuncture was compared to treading the edge of a precipice.

These people were somehow aware of the rhythms of the body that we now know to be part of our physiology. There was a deep conviction that it was no use giving treatment, and particularly acupuncture, unless one took account of body rhythms. We now know that there is indeed a twenty-four hour rhythm. This, as mentioned earlier, is known as Circadian rhythm. The monthly period in women is governed by endocrine glandular changes under the control of the brain. It may or may not be, in turn, in synchrony with the lunar cycle, but it has always seemed to me to be more than coincidence that both are normally twenty-eight day cycles. There may be other cycles to which we respond to unconsciously, such as the seasons of the year. We know that certain conditions are more common in spring and fall, two seasons that appear to be more stressful to many people, although this is not the conventional explanation.

Public health statistics tell us, for example, that there is a slightly increased incidence of leukemia in the spring.

An early tract was written by Hsu about 930 A.D. on how to select loci for acupuncture or moxibustion according to the diurnal cycle, the day of the month, and the season of the year. They were aware of the circulation of the blood, describing "the flow in the tract and channel runs on and on, and never stops; a ceaseless movement in an annular circuit." This was stated in the second century B.C. and Harvey's discovery of the circulation of blood was hailed as a brand new discovery when his findings were published in 1628.

Unfortunately, although all of this arose from true observation and instinctive knowledge, the structure became so complex that the ordinary practitioner could only learn it by rote and in the end, it became arbitrary and mechanical, dissolving into ritual, as happens in religious rites. The question for us today, of course, is whether acupuncture or pulse diagnosis fit in any way into our present knowledge of the functions of the body. Modern experiments have been tried on animals. It was found in dogs that inflammation, caused by introduction of bacteria, could be partially inhibited by acupuncture. But, if a particular segment of the sympathetic chain was removed, the protective effect was lost. The sympathetic chain is part of the autonomic nervous system that we will be considering in more detail later. Suffice it to say here that this nervous system is controlled by a part of the brain that is not under voluntary control. It has also been found that acupuncture gives rise to the release of endorphins in the brain. These important substances, that were discovered recently, have very important effects in the brain that lead to relief of pain. There is, therefore, a logical explanation for acupuncture as a treatment. It is interesting that Sir William Osler, one of the great clinicians of the 20th century, wrote in his textbook *Principles and Practice of Medicine* that acupuncture was, in acute cases, the most efficient treatment for lumbago, or as it is known today, chronic back strain.

Derrick Lonsdale M.D.

Stress In Disease

Hans Selye, the investigator of stress on animals, wrote that "research on stress will be most fruitful if it is guided by the theory that we must learn to imitate the body's own autopharmacological efforts to combat the stress factors in disease." Thus, the dynamic equilibrium that was epitomized in yin and yang has been considered the balance of health in the eyes of many an ancient and traditional physician through the ages. Today, we are able to recognize that this physiologic balance is maintained by a computer in the brain, sending messages to the organs of the body via the autonomic nervous system and the collection of internal glands known as the endocrine system.

Now that we know more about the body machinery we can make sense from data that was originally collected by observation. It enables us to understand mental as well as physical imbalance; that the brain and body must be in balance when the organism is at rest; and that imbalance is a temporary phenomenon that enables us to react to environmental "stress." If a temporary imbalance that, under normal circumstances expresses an emotional state appropriately, becomes excessively exaggerated in response to a stress stimulus, it becomes abnormal. The observations and philosophy of ancient China help us today to understand the real nature of health and disease.

The teachings of Hippocrates fit in easily with the concepts of ancient China. He taught rest, diet, and "anti-stress" as the foundation of treatment. He encouraged the body to become well by simply taking it out of commission for a while and letting it heal itself. The quality of diet was the most important thing that people could do for themselves. Our medical complex has built up a terrifying structure that really encourages illness to thrive rather than reversing it. People have been led to see their illnesses in diagnostic compartments, often with Latin names, where each is catalogued and considered as a separate entity. A modern physician does not have the power of a witch doctor who is seen by his unsophisticated patient as having special powers. If the modern physician tells a patient that he has to start healing himself by following the proper rules of nutrition, the credibility gap is apt to be unbridgeable.

Medical school professors teach their students contemporary beliefs and they have accepted the rules of the day as the truth. They may have invested huge sums of money in equipment that is considered to be the "state of the art," and it is not likely that they wish to hear that another approach is necessary. Hippocrates is thought to have done the best thing that he could under the primitive circumstances that existed in his day. Complementary Alternative Medicine is seeking to put the clock forward by improving on the present form of mainstream medicine. Surgery, skilful and dramatic as it is, is often an admission of medical failure. It is not the best outcome to require organs to be removed because they are damaged beyond repair. Admittedly, this is frequently life saving but it is "shutting the stable door after the horse has gone." The problem is what caused the organs to become sick in the first place. Antibiotics should be reserved for life threatening situations caused by microorganisms that are sensitive to their effects. The body is a self-repairing machine that heals itself. All that it needs is the right "fuel" to provide the necessary energy.

Cause of Disease

During the Dark Ages the cause of disease was unknown. The discovery of microorganisms gradually ushered in the antibiotic age, but Louis Pasteur, who made the original discoveries, had an extremely hard time getting them accepted as a cause of disease. The dramatic thought change required was too stressful to the majority of his peers and, as usual in these circumstances, automatically triggered anger. This is occurring today in the introduction of Complementary Alternative Medicine (CAM). Anger is generated in the minds of orthodox medical practitioners and is predictable. It is no different from that which held back the progress anticipated by the discoveries of Pasteur. "Turf" battles will have to be fought, but it will be the consumer who ultimately makes the decisions. The public is more and more accepting of the principles that are being defined by CAM. Unfortunately this will take time since the profession is controlled by the drug and insurance industries.

After the invention of the microscope, it was possible to see individual cells and the fingerprints of disease became known by the changes seen in affected cells. This discovery has misled us in our quest for appropriate approaches to disease. The prevailing attitude has remained that we must kill the microorganism. It has been reported that Pasteur, on his deathbed, said that the "terrain was more important." By that, he was indicating that he was of the opinion that the attacking germ was less important than the mechanisms of defense used by the body. With the exception of infections, where a battle is joined between the attacking microorganism and the patient, we now have compelling reasons to believe that all ongoing disease is caused by biochemical abnormality within the cells. Disease might be compared with a storm passing through a geographical area, leaving in its wake the damage that can be observed long after the storm has passed. The analogy for the disease is the storm, whereas the damage that is observed afterwards is the analogy for what the pathologist sees with his microscope. We need to assist the natural healing process and this cannot be done with pharmaceutical drugs. The only way to assist the natural process of repair is through the use of nutrients that provide the cells with the additional energy required to initiate healing.

We need to kill the invading microorganism if it can be done without damaging the defensive mechanisms of the affected patient. Antibiotics are life-saving weapons in many situations that might otherwise be lethal. They have, however, become a staple method of treating some conditions that do not require them and produce damaging effects that could be avoidable.

They are "two-edged swords." Penicillin was the first drug that could kill a microorganism with what initially appeared to be complete safety to the patient. Sensitivity to it has, however, killed a relatively small number of people since its inception. Nevertheless, people with pneumonia and other infections, who had previously died from the onslaught of a microorganism that could not be saved by ordinary means, became well almost immediately. The discovery had a downside- bacteria underwent mutation that made them resistant to one antibiotic after another. Our attention has been fixed on attempts to find ways and means of safely killing infectious organisms without giving consideration to how we can help the normal body defenses. The idea of "killing the enemy" spread to attempts to kill viruses, unfortunately lacking in effectiveness. It also spread to the field of cancer where we are still trying to find the ideal drug that will be lethal to the cancer cell without being lethal to the patient. The "War on Cancer" has largely failed, though billions of dollars have been poured into this type of research. The drugs that are used are appallingly toxic and most patients feel very ill indeed from the treatment. In fact in many cases it is the treatment that kills the patient, not the disease.

    The situation is parallel to that faced by farmers in their war on destructive insects. The insects become genetically mutated, like the bacteria, and become resistant to the current chemical in use. They too have become more and more toxic to the humans that consume the agricultural products and we now have thousands of such chemicals that are polluting earth rapidly, to the ultimate cost of all animal life, as well as our own. By altering the natural balance ordained by Mother Nature, we are interfering with the intricate web of life by which the plant and animal kingdoms are inextricably related. It is obviously destructive and, for the most part, is either going unheeded by the majority of people, or is presenting problems that are impossible to solve. One has only to pick up the monthly issues of *National Geographic* to see how this is affecting the world that supports our life and every creature on it. The term "endangered species" appears regularly in the pages of this magazine.

A Paradigm Shift

The shift in medical thinking needs to be towards the self-healing powers of the body and not to "control" the disease as the present system attempts. When an orthopedist tackles a fractured bone, he is a technician. He has to line up the fragments in a mechanical sense. It is the bone that heals itself. We can help this process by making sure that the cells necessary to perform this task have enough energy.

The modern physician has been taught to have faith in the wonders of the pharmacy and drugs are produced in a bewildering and confusing array, each covered by a patent that gives exclusive sales for a number of years. The tests required by the Federal Drug Agency in order to get a drug approved amount to hundreds of millions of dollars passed on to the consumer. Often a drug under a given trade name may be prescribed simply because a physician has been able to remember that particular name, derived from advertising The *Physicians' Desk Reference* gets bigger each year that it is published, together with additional supplements that may follow. It becomes virtually impossible to keep track of the indications and still more difficult for busy practitioners to keep up with the potential side effects of each.

A drug might be defined as a substance that affects the physiology of the body. Nutrients also do this by providing the energy required for each cell to function. When they are ingested in high doses, however, they act as drugs because their action is to stimulate physiology to a higher degree. The first thing that the body does with a pharmaceutical is to recognize it as a foreigner and to break it down to its metabolic byproducts. It recognizes a vitamin as a nutrient that fits in with its physiology. If used as a drug in this way, it has to be in an effective dose and can be toxic if that dose is increased to excess, the yin and yang. Mother Nature provided an adequate supply of these chemical substances that enabled the development of the animal kingdom.

The mental state in disease is as important as the physical state. A witch doctor has the power to kill or cure, simply by placing or removing a curse from the victim. A young African native had been told by the tribal witch doctor that he would die after a curse was placed on him. The victim languished and began attending the modern western styled medical clinic that existed in the locality. Every up-to-date means that was available was used, to no effect. Finally, the clinic requested that the witch doctor remove the curse and forgive his victim, whereupon the young man began instantly to recover. It was the implicit faith of the victim in the absolute power of the witch doctor that was the key. We do not understand the mechanism, known as the placebo effect.

In any drug trial there will be a certain number of subjects in the study who will be better in health from the placebo. It depends solely on the faith factor of the individual. If the unknown treatment is placebo and the subject believes that it is the real thing, it will work for that person. It is this factor that has given rise to the gold standard of drug testing, the double-blind placebo-controlled study. The subjects do not know whether they are in the placebo group or the drug test group and neither does the investigator or anyone who has contact with them. This is because the outcome in a test subject can be influenced unconsciously by someone who knows which group that subject is in. The decision as to whether the drug has a greater effect than the placebo depends upon whether there is a statistically significant difference between the two groups. The faith factor can work both ways, for benefit or for regression.

The late Norman Cousins told of his experience in hospital when he was being treated for a disease that usually cripples its victims. He noted that pessimism and negative thoughts could do harm, so why not try to reverse that scenario. He obtained permission to have comical movies introduced into his room, and after a good laugh he found that he could get some sleep without a pain-killer. This approach, together with injections of Vitamin C, resulted in his cure.

It is, therefore extremely important for a physician to provide a patient with a positive signal that the outcome is a return to health. In the modern world of medicine, this is extremely difficult to do. Physicians no longer have any kind of "guru" power over the patient. They are considered to be well-educated people with all the fallibility of anyone else. The witch doctor depends upon the unsophisticated faith of the patient in witchcraft. It works because it is the power within the mind of the patient who heals himself. An adverse effect can be produced by negative suggestion, the principle behind "voodoo." Science and technology have come to replace the faith factor because we believe that these wonders are able to find out what is wrong quickly, precisely, and accurately. Today, the diagnosis heard by the patient may easily result in a sense of hopelessness that has its own adverse effect.

There is a wide gap between the technological methods of detecting the fingerprints of disease and the ability to treat it. For a disease, such as cancer, it is the first strike against the patient's ability to help himself through the power of his own mind. The diagnosis becomes a potential death sentence. True faith is a rarity but it is the principle that governs success in Christian Science. We can easily give lip service to the idea of faith, but skepticism reverses its effect.

I met a gentleman who told me that he had cured himself of cancer, using the macrobiotic diet. He impressed me because there was no hint of surprise that the diet had worked. He was completely convinced that it was the only way to treat cancer and I wondered whether it was his faith that was as important as the diet. In our hunt for the magic bullets of science, we have forgotten that the body has its own healing powers and can generate them when the mind is positively concentrated on the

A Nutritional Approach to a Revised Model for Medicine

problem. It matters little what the focal point of faith is. Surely, it is this simple fact that has given rise to the diversity of religions.

Perhaps research into the pathways of the brain will gradually solve the mystery. My hypothesis is that the belief factor concentrates the mind on the part of the body that requires extra attention in order to start the healing process. If it requires extra energy to do this, perhaps the resources of the body have to be husbanded and focused at the point of most concern. This is why I have often thought that nutrition has simply "discovered" the mechanism of the placebo effect by providing the extra energy that is required. I consider that the nutrients, by providing this extra energy for cellular function, result in a marked increase in efficiency over and above that required for ordinary daily function. Perhaps it can be considered a revival; a renaissance of the approach to healing that was advised and practiced by Hippocrates.

We have mastered revival in an emergency that would have spelled certain death a few years ago. Surgery has advanced to a point of extraordinary skill, but both are spawned by failure to prevent the crisis from occurring in the first place. With the exception of trauma and congenital defects in anatomical development, surgery may one day be minimized. It has been published that thirty-six percent of admissions to a university hospital were conditions that were actually produced by physicians. They were not failures of treatment, but actively caused by it.

I was a member of the staff of a large multi-disciplined clinic. One day, on ward rounds, a resident was reporting the findings in the case of an adolescent boy. He outlined the history as usual and then went through all the tests to which the patient had been subjected. Each one was described as negative and when he came to the end of his description, there was a pause before the staff member spoke. As we moved away from the bed he finally said, "Well, I really thought that there was something wrong with that boy." It clearly expressed the prevailing attitude toward psychosomatic illness. The point is that the boy's symptoms were considered to be fake. A "functional" condition is referred to a psychiatrist or psychologist. This form of disease is the commonest of all and has more to do with diet than psychology. It may sometimes be the forerunner of organic disease and is a true marker of the decline in health that we are seeing in our society.

CHAPTER 3

THE BRAIN CONTAINS A COMPUTER

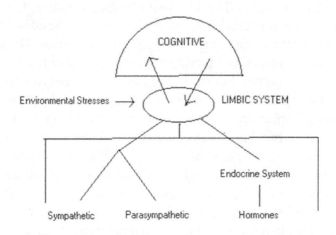

FIGURE 1: Diagrammatic representation of brain/body model

A Revised Paradigm Shift In Thinking

In chapter two the present disease model described is that of "killing the enemy," whereas the model described here pays much more attention to the way we adapt to the various environmental stimuli encountered on a day-to-day basis throughout life. Understanding the development of Complementary Alternative Medicine requires a paradigm shift in thinking.

Figure 1 represents the simplest presentation of this model. Although we each have only one brain anatomically, it is divided conceptually into two functional sections. Figure 1 does not take anatomy or structure into consideration.

Freud recognized the subconscious mind, but did not understand that it was really a computer since computers had not been invented at that time. The cognitive or conscious mind is still poorly understood, although great strides have been made in research. We do not understand completely the mechanism of intelligence and there is some doubt as to whether we can truly exercise "free will," defined as possessing an ability to take complete control over all our conscious actions, make choices, or change our minds. The alternative to that, of course, is the idea that the brain is a "black box" which arranges all the complexities of human behavior at a highly organized reflex level. The expert neurologists presently studying the brain deny that the cognitive brain is a computer, but the lower brain works below conscious level and computer seems to be the logical explanation of its function. Sanity and rational behavior is a complex dialogue between the two brains. The lines drawn between the cognitive brain and the computer in Figure 1 represent the continuous communication that goes on between the two at all times when we are conscious. The lines drawn between the "autonomic" and "endocrine" systems, body organs, and the computer represent the dialogue that must exist between them throughout life. This is the brain/body machinery that enables us to adapt to the constant environmental changes that we encounter.

In the newborn infant the lower brain is the functional one and the cognitive, although anatomically present, is not. Thus, we have no conscious awareness at birth. We have a computer that is programmed, enabling us to cry, to be soothed, to express anger by the nature of the cry and express all the limited emotional reactions of such an infant. The newborn, at this stage, is purely automatic, because the connections have not yet been completely hardwired. Whether he feels pain in the same way as an older child or not is a moot point. He certainly cries in response to painful stimulus, but it is probably purely reflex.

A Nutritional Approach to a Revised Model for Medicine

It may well be "remembered" in the form of a "file" incorporated into the "hard drive" of the computer. This is probably the way that something as devastating as child abuse is retained. It is never erased as a "file" and will continue to interfere with the normal dialogue between the two brains throughout life.

It is important to remember that our perception of the world depends upon all sensory input that is interpreted by the brain. If those mechanisms of interpretation are immature, non-functional, or distorted, the interpretation will be abnormal. Philosophers throughout the ages have asked whether the world in which we live is really there. At first sight, this seems to be absurd but we "see, hear, smell, and touch" the world in which we live and our perception of it depends upon how it is interpreted in our brains. The body is nothing without the brain.

The infant urinates and defecates into his diaper and has no conscious awareness of the act. These are functions that will be overridden later by the cognitive brain when a dialogue has been established. As this awareness develops, it is a process of biochemical and electrical maturation and has little to do with so-called toilet training. Of course, the growing child is introduced to the toilet as the proper place and becomes aware of its use. But it is strictly a developmental phenomenon and would take place in any normal child, whether toilet training is instituted or not.

Occasionally, an infant is born with a normal looking head but the only brain within it is the brain stem. If a light is placed behind the infant's head, it will glow because it contains only the guidance system that we are referring to as the computer. The rest of the space in the skull is taken up with fluid. It is, of course, incompatible with ultimate survival. The initial impression is that the infant is quite normal. He looks normal and he cries. He will suck from a bottle or the breast and he can be soothed. His brain contains the machinery that presides over purely reflex function but it has no capacity at all for the maturation required to grow towards childhood and adult status. After a short while, it becomes obvious that there is no further development and the infant must eventually die.

During the first six months of life, brain growth in the human is phenomenal and this is best seen by examining an infant head circumference chart as used in a pediatrician's office. The growth is exponential and the curve of the chart is almost vertical initially, gradually sloping off to the age of about six months. During the second six months the slope is quite gradual. The increase in head circumference is closely related to the growth of the brain as its complexity increases. Brain cells increase in number and become more specialized. Increasingly complex electro-chemical reactions and cell specialization form the basis of maturation. One day, this sophistication reaches a point when a message coming into the computer from the bladder is passed on to the cognitive brain. In effect, a dialogue begins between the two brains and the higher brain is being asked, "What shall we do about this message from the bladder?" The answer is dependent upon whether the infant has been introduced to the practical use of a toilet, and whether maturation has proceeded far enough to inhibit the normal reflex that would be initiated by the computer. It is failure of this maturation that is responsible for bed wetting (enuresis).

The more primitive lower brain dominates function in a young child and it is obviously important to understand the gradual electro-chemical process by which more and more advisory action is required from the cognitive. It is amazingly similar to the increasing complexity that is introduced into a man-made computer as more and more software programs are added to the hard drive.

The Computer

Calling part of the brain a computer appears to conflict with the philosophical notions of the "spirit" and the "soul." People say that there has got to be more to humanity than whirling electrons and complex chemical reactions. There is no practical evidence for the existence of either the soul or the spirit. Philosophers have used them to explain much that we do not know about ourselves, dismissing them as that part of a dying person that flees the body toward a new life. The role of a physician as a teacher, however, is to try to get his patient to understand the fundamentals of brain/body machinery that has to be serviced to maintain mental and physical health.

The limbic system brain is a complex computer that reacts to input stimulus. It is constantly receiving all the communication signals from both the outside environment and from the body. The "personality" of an individual is partly inherited and partly programmed by upbringing and experience. Emotional reactions will be predictable, to a large degree, by understanding the nature of this personality, but it is not a thinking process. It is an automated, biochemically driven reaction to a stimulus and we are all programmed to react in a similar way to a given stimulus. For example, we smile in response to a pleasant stimulus and frown when it is unpleasant. If a person receives a telegram giving bad news, the computerized reaction is a predictable emotion. This is the result of a chemical reaction in the computer. The conscious brain can override the "commands" of the computer for a lot of our behavior. This, however, means that there has to be an appropriate dialogue between them. For example, although breathing is a purely automatic process, governed by the computer, we can override it voluntarily, requiring an effort of will that is determined by the cognitive. When we are asleep, the automatic control mechanisms must take over this vital process. If it becomes dysfunctional, as happens when the electrochemical mechanisms in the brain stem are affected, breathing is compromised and we get sleep apnea, a common problem in the world of today. Sudden Infant Death Syndrome (SIDS), also still too common, is in the same category and could easily be prevented by understanding and using what we know about the chemistry related to energy metabolism in those vitally important brain cells.

Derrick Lonsdale M.D.

Emotions, governed automatically by the limbic brain, result from various stimuli and are associated with predictable reflex changes of a physical nature in the body. For example, anger will be associated with a typical facial expression and other changes by which we can observe it in an affected person. Such complex reactions are built into our genetic makeup and the pattern of associated behavior is appropriate. It is not a thinking process and it is maintained by normal brain chemistry. It is modified by properly introduced training and experience that might be compared with the addition of software to a computer.

We know, for instance, that our assumed gender roles are programmed into us within the first two years of life. It is taken for granted that a person with male genitalia is to be raised as a boy and one with female genitalia as a girl. It is possible, however, to raise a normal boy as a girl and vice versa, simply by training the individual to assume the gender role. Such a role-training is entered into the "hard drive" as a permanent "file" and cannot be erased after the second year of life.

Laughter is appropriate under predictable conditions, but an abnormal response is inappropriate as in the case of a man recorded in medical literature who would begin to laugh helplessly when having sexual intercourse. Abnormal chemistry gives rise to abnormal behavior. Both mental and physical stimulation are forms of "stress" and our adaptive responses are automated, but can be modified cognitively. Thinking and conscious awareness are much more complicated phenomena, about which we know very little as yet. Computer scientists are, however, trying to build a robot with artificial intelligence, implying that it may be possible for a man-made computer to perform in an intelligent manner and to make choices if enough complexity is introduced.

Certainly, an important function of the cognitive or conscious brain is to advise the more primitive brain computer that an action is permissible within the confines of contemporary society. When the dialogue between the two is functioning normally, we have sanity, but when the computer "takes over command" it exposes the primitive person within each one of us. The resulting behavior may be irrational to observers but not necessarily to the perpetrator, potentially important in trying to understand behavior like violent crime and vandalism. The cognitive brain may be aware of the action, but powerless to stop it.

If it can be proved in an Ohio court that a crime was committed by someone who knew what he was doing but was powerless to stop, it can come under the heading of "temporary insanity." This is extremely difficult to prove, particularly in our present attitude toward crime being considered to be a purely voluntary act that must be punished.

"Blind anger" or "seeing red" may be a real phenomenon. Perhaps a person can become so berserk that he can commit a violent crime without cognitive awareness. There is a precedent in the so-called Twinkie case, tried in California. A man committed murder and his defense rested on the plea that his criminal act was brought about by the state of his brain induced from a craving for that particular commercial brand of sweets. One cannot help wondering whether the murders alleged to have been committed by O.J. were performed in a state of blind anger. Could it be that such a person is so deranged at the time of the crime that he actually did not know that he was committing it? If it were so, he would have been "insane" at the moment of the crime. One also wonders whether he consumed a great deal of the soft drink that he advertized on television commercials.

This may seem to be too far fetched, but as an example, sleep walking is an extremely complex act while maintaining unconsciousness. It would have to be shown that the brain was in a state of biochemical abnormality and that it could slip back into a normal state of balance (*homeostasis*) afterwards. Homeostasis is the intermediate state of mind between two extremes of possible behavior, perhaps fury on the one side and exaggerated tranquility on the other. Depression is one extreme and euphoria the other, the personality characterized by Pagliacci and known to be the behavioral characteristics of many comedians. We might say that homeostasis is the correct mixture of yin and yang while at rest.

The limbic system computer might be compared with a radio. The incoming sensory input is data processed and the reflex emotional state and actions induced. On completion the brain approaches an intermediate state of balance. If the volume control on a radio is increased to an extreme, it becomes an unpleasant experience for the listener. Could it be that the mechanisms of violence in human brains are dependent on "volume" of input and the threshold of limbic system reaction? High calorie malnutrition, particularly the ingestion of simple carbohydrates, certainly induces a lower threshold of reaction by the limbic system and the emotional reactions are increased in volume. Whether it can overwhelm the cognitive supervision to the point of violence is unknown, but temper tantrums in children are exaggerated by high calorie malnutrition and they can quite commonly be associated with minor acts of violence, such as kicking a wall.

Turning back to the process of thinking as performed by the cognitive brain, it is possibly brought about by a mass of reflexes that connect and deliver an eventual conclusion that reaches a new plane of understanding.

It might be illustrated by the persistence of Edison when he tested thousands of materials that would glow with sufficient brilliance to shed light when an electric current was passed through it. There was a logical sequence in the brain reactions that we might identify as thought. We know also that some very complex problems have been solved by a person when asleep. A scientist goes to bed with the problem "on his mind" and awakens with the solution. It is as though the brain works on its own and that is really not any different from putting complex information into a mainframe computer which "data processes" it and arrives at a solution.

The Hypothalamic, Autonomic, Endocrine Axis

The autonomic nervous system is like a double channel telephone line to every organ in the body. The endocrine system is a group of glands. Each gland releases its particular hormone or hormones into the blood stream on receipt of an executive signal from the computer and their concentrations are controlled by biofeedback. It is difficult for us to imitate this natural action by the administration of artificially created hormones. They function as messengers to body cells to stimulate action, contributing to the total activity of the whole organism. Like rockets sent out from earth to dock with a satellite, hormones have to "dock" with receptors on the surface of cells. A message passes into the cell through its surrounding membrane and this stimulates machinery within the cell.

The autonomic nervous system is controlled automatically by the limbic computer and works by balanced action of the sympathetic and parasympathetic branches. Like yin and yang, one does the opposite of the other. For example, the sympathetic branch is the "action system" and is used to accelerate the heart. When fully activated it governs the fight-or-flight survival reflex. The parasympathetic decelerates the heart and might be called the "rest and be thankful system." Thus, fine control of heart speed is maintained and a person who is at rest should have a heart rate that is intermediate between fast and slow, the so-called resting pulse. Their relationship is an ever-shifting one in the continuous process of adaptation. Dominance of either one is temporary under normal circumstances to guide a given adaptive response, but when the action is completed, the two systems must go back into a state of balance known as homeostasis.

The neurotransmitters used by the nervous system are chemicals synthesized in the body and are energy transducers, meaning that they function by inducing electrical energy. Thus, signals to body organs that initiate action, are a combination of chemical and electrical energy. To illustrate this, the electric eel is capable of producing a powerful electrical shock to stun or kill its prey. The organ that performs this is an adaptation of a nerve. The brain of the animal releases a signal through this nerve, but the terminal end of the nerve, known as a *synaptosome*, is grossly enlarged, extending from the head to the tail. Evolution has caused this part of the nerve to become an electrical condenser. Chemical energy is released into the synaptosome from a neurotransmitter. Thus, a nervous message, generated in the brain of the eel is used to kill or stun prey with a bolt of static electricity.

The principles of this nervous mechanism in the eel apply to our own nervous system. Electrical energy is generated in synaptosomes that are not enlarged like those of the eel and the electrical energy is in microvolts. There is an essential "oneness" throughout the animal kingdom, a fact that we seem to be ignoring more and more.

Consciousness

We must conclude that nothing happens in the body without the brain computer being involved. The brain "talks" to the body in a chemical/electrical language. Messengers enable body organs to "talk" to each other and back to the brain. The limbic brain is sometimes called the reptilian system, because that is virtually all that a reptile possesses. Thus, a reptile may have no conscious awareness, more like a living robot. As the complexity of the animal kingdom increased through the continued experiment of evolution, the question arose, when did the phenomenon of consciousness begin? We do not know whether we are the only animal on earth that has conscious awareness. It may be that this is only possible with a certain degree of complexity of brain construction, although there is no clear indication of what degree is required.

We can perform very complex actions while unconscious, as in sleep walking. All the primitive, life-preserving mechanisms are controlled by the brain computer during sleep. When we are conscious, the two components of the brain work together and we can use conscious control over some of these functions, as in the example of breathing.

In Greek mythology, there is a play called "Ondine's Curse," a story that has recurred down through the ages in various forms, so it is undoubtedly a reflection of a clinical observation with an explanation invented through lack of understanding. Ondine was a water nymph who was jilted by her human lover. In return, she cursed him with the loss of all automatically controlled functions in his body. He had to remain conscious in order to run his body mechanisms, including breathing. Eventually, of course, he had to sleep and that caused him to die in his sleep.

There is a disease called Ondine's Curse in which something goes wrong with the automatic breathing apparatus in the brain computer. The patient literally "forgets to breathe." I have had some experience with this disease in a girl who periodically stopped breathing for no obvious reason. I remember seeing her sitting on the side of her hospital bed. Her hands were raised in front of her, her eyes were staring and wide open and she was blue from deficiency of oxygen delivered to the tissues. She admitted to an extreme sense of panic, just as any of us would experience if breathing were to be obstructed. But we would also be struggling to get that life preserving breath, whereas this girl did not know why she felt this way and was making no effort to get the breath that her brain was failing to tell her that she needed. A sense of panic is a sensory phenomenon caused by the build-up of carbon dioxide and lack of oxygen in the brain. There is a center in the brain stem that is part of the computer. It is this center which initiates powerful efforts to suck in the air that is needed under such circumstances, as for example in drowning. In this girl, that center was damaged and she failed to recognize the necessity to take the needed breath. When I administered oxygen with a mask, the blue color of her skin, termed *cyanosis*, cleared up. The sense of panic disappeared and that look of pure fright, represented by the staring eyes and characteristic appearance that we can all recognize, also disappeared.

She had to "remember" to do this normally automatic function. But another part of the computer registered the panic that is an accompanying feature of suffocation without her being able to understand the reason for her sensations, thus demonstrating that the damage was affecting the respiratory center exclusively. It reminds us that we survive in a hostile environment because our brain/body "machinery" enables us to adapt to the kaleidoscope of physical changes that we encounter throughout our lives. The computer is stimulated by visual, olfactory, auditory, and tactile input that all have to be data processed. It must react also to abstract perceptions such as a verbal insult. Because of the program written into the "hard drive," there is instantaneous recognition of threat or danger, inducing survival reflexes. Upbringing, training, and experience can modify our reactions.

The Limbic System Is A Conductor to Orchestrate Environmental Adaptation

The body can be compared with an orchestra. The organs represent a bank of instrumentalists with cells that represent musicians. Under the "baton" of a brain "conductor," the "symphony of health" results. No orchestra could survive without a conductor. Thus, the symphony can be destroyed because an instrument fails or, perhaps more threateningly, because the conductor fails. The commonest health breakdown in Americans today is because of chemical damage to the computer. The easiest way to induce this damage is to indulge in "high calorie malnutrition." It is dangerous because we are unable to perceive its effects in ourselves. Its results are essentially those of disorganized adaptive responses, including emotional reactions that are released much too easily. The computer becomes excitable and over-reacts to incoming stimuli. It is not that the reactions are in and of themselves abnormal. They are merely grossly exaggerated as in the analogy of the radio.

Beriberi Is the Prototype for High Calorie Malnutrition

High calorie malnutrition is a scourge of immense proportions since the consumption of sugar in its many different forms is actively encouraged. My realization and education came from studying the average diet of my young patients. The cardinal case that I described in some detail in my book *Why I Left Orthodox Medicine* was a six-year-old boy whose neurological illness occurred intermittently. Each episode of his illness was an exact imitation of beriberi. Because of this, Vitamin B1 was administered but he did not respond clinically until the dose had become huge. Later studies performed at the National Institutes of Health were able to show that he had a genetically determined weakness in the energy-yielding mechanism that uses Vitamin B1. We now recognize that such a person is "vitamin dependent" rather than a simple dietary deficiency. This child required from 300 to 600 milligrams of thiamine a day in order to prevent the recurrent neurological episodes. The recommended normal daily dose of this vitamin is about 1.5 milligrams a day.

The case of this child made me begin a library research into every aspect of beriberi and its known association with this vitamin. In experimenting with the administration of vitamins, particularly thiamine, I discovered that a surprisingly large number of children with diseases that were considered to be untreatable, would respond, at least partially, to vitamin therapy. Within a few years, I had completely transformed my viewpoint about what I was doing as a physician.

I came across several papers that had been long forgotten in the medical library and which, if one knew how to fit them to clinical problems of today, made perfect sense. The most important revelations came from a discovery that the brain stem computer becomes much more reactive when it is insulted by a deficiency of Vitamin B1. A greater degree of metabolic inefficiency makes it less and less sensitive and eventually destroys it if the malnutrition is severe enough. It enabled me to understand why infantile beriberi caused a death in infants which was an exact facsimile of crib death, or Sudden Infant Death Syndrome (SIDS). What was perhaps much more profound, was that I found beriberi, in its early stages, causes dominant functional imbalance in either the sympathetic or the parasympathetic arms of the autonomic nervous system. The general term that is applied to this is what I call *Functional Dysautonomia,* meaning that functions applied to this automatic nervous system are deranged, not because of structural disease, but because of inefficient biochemistry in the cells of the brain where the control mechanisms exist.

The traditional explanation for beriberi is Vitamin B1 deficiency. But I also discovered that the early investigators of nutrient deficiency diseases in the 1930s were certain that beriberi and pure thiamine deficiency were not the same. Although it is unnecessary to go into details about the differences, beriberi is an example of prolonged high calorie malnutrition, although Vitamin B1 deficiency is a vital component. It is still relevant today, mainly in rice eating cultures. Our food must consist of fuel that, when burned (oxidized) yields energy. It must contain vitamins and minerals that "ignite" it and control the resultant energy. The third component is oxygen and all three must be present in a proper balance.

High calorie malnutrition has its effect on the brain computer. The analogy of a choked engine in a car is the equivalent in the human body, particularly in the brain and heart where oxygen consumption is heaviest. The fuel, being oxidized inefficiently, gives rise to various forms of acid which are the equivalent of the black smoke in the exhaust pipe of a car when the engine is choked. These acids are excreted from the body in urine.

I have looked for these acids in neurological conditions in children and have often found them to be present. Many of them were in hospital with traditional disease diagnoses. This often means that little or nothing is known of the underlying mechanisms. What it seems to represent is inefficient chemistry in the brain and nervous system. Some of them improved by trying the harmless experiment of vitamin therapy. Thiamine was often a most important one to use, probably reflecting the use of simple carbohydrates in the diet. So how does abnormal biochemistry in the limbic brain become translated into a variety of clinical conditions that include all kinds of "emotional" changes?

Limbic System Disease

Marginally inefficient metabolism in the limbic system causes it to over-react to incoming stimuli, not under-react. Although this is the exact opposite of what might be expected, loss of function gradually follows if the metabolism becomes even more degraded. It might be that this over-reaction in a mild state of inefficiency is protective. If a person is sleeping in a room that is gradually filling with carbon dioxide it would be an obvious survival advantage for an alarm to be triggered in the brain that would cause awakening. In the early stages it would create an inefficient metabolic situation similar to marginal vitamin deficiency or lack of oxygen, acting as a warning. High calorie malnutrition, resulting in marginally inefficient metabolism, stimulates the alarm system. Automatic survival reflexes, for example the fight-or-flight (panic attacks), become more easily activated and exaggerated. The limbic system does not think. It reacts according to the way that it is programmed. If its reflex reactions are exaggerated it is not, in and of itself, abnormal. It is merely a "high volume" response. There is a threshold of reaction to any given stimulus and high calorie malnutrition lowers the threshold. The response might be seen as merely an exaggeration of what the person might do under normal circumstances.

Our ancestors depended on the fight-or-flight reflex for survival in a dangerous environment. Our genetic inheritance is the same but the environment is different. For a cave man, confronted with the vision of a saber-toothed tiger, a fight-or-flight reflex was potentially life saving. The emotional and physiological changes that occur are mediated through the release of hormones in the endocrine system and through messages to the sympathetic arm of the autonomic nervous system. All of them can be seen as preparation for action.

Panic attacks, sometimes nocturnal, are commonly experienced by many people today, triggered by a dysfunctional limbic system giving rise to an unnecessary survival reflex. A trivial sensory input such as a change in barometric pressure may be enough to fire it because the threshold of reaction in the limbic system has been lowered. By far the commonest cause is high calorie malnutrition.

A typical example was that of a six-year-old boy. He was one of four children, all of whom were carriers of a genetically determined disease that required two copies of the gene to express the disease. The father had the disease and his children were all obligate carriers of one copy of the gene. It has long been considered that a person with a carrier state of this type would be totally unaffected by it and be in perfect health. In this family, none of the four children were ever well, but none of them had the symptoms of the disease like the father. They all became easily angered and fatigued and their symptoms, while not amounting to any specific indicator of the disease in the father, were quite diverse and different in the children.

It became clear to me that each of them was really suffering from a lack of cellular energy and each was helped by paying attention to their nutrition and vitamin supplements. The boy had a strange story. He had been described as "very grown up" and was considered to be emotionally stable and secure for his age. He had to visit a dentist and the visit turned out to be extremely traumatic. The dentist even had to chase him and bring him back

A Nutritional Approach to a Revised Model for Medicine

to the dental chair, suggesting that the child had a fight-or-flight reflex

After this visit, his personality changed abruptly. He became afraid of everything, needed a night light in his bedroom, became very insecure and whined constantly. The parents emphasized that this was a very dramatic and sudden change, clearly related to the dental examination. I merely changed his high calorie malnutrition and gave him some supplementary vitamins. They included Vitamin B1 since a blood test had shown that he was deficient in this vitamin. There was a slow change back to his former secure personality. Traditionally, it would have been seen as a psychological problem. Although the dentist was the stressor, it was the exaggerated reaction of the child's limbic system that caused the abrupt change in behavior because his metabolic state was poised on the brink of inefficiency.

Another example was a woman who had been crying night and day for three weeks. Virtually anything would start her off and she would cry and scream in high volume. Her family had unanimously voted to send her for psychiatric examination and possible admission to a mental disease hospital. She had no idea of why she behaved in this manner and her relatives thought that she was "crazy" when she insisted on obtaining nutritional treatment. She was treated with a series of intravenously administered vitamin and mineral supplements. Not only did she become completely normal in every way, she turned out to be an exceptionally intelligent woman and returned to her life in a renewed state. It had been seen by her relatives as a "nervous breakdown."

If symptoms are associated with a series of normal laboratory studies, modern mainstream medicine would call it "functional," a word that has become synonymous with neurotic or psychosomatic. The patient may be given a "tranquilizer" that eases symptoms without addressing their cause. Caffeine, however, stimulates the limbic system and is often one of the drugs that may be responsible. The only way to find whether this is true is to discontinue coffee and see if it makes a difference. Chocolate, sweets, soft drinks (particularly those containing aspartame), fruit juice, milk (yes milk!) are frequently causative also. Skepticism is usually generated and the dialogue that follows represents a "mental gradient" that has to be climbed by the counselor. I spend about seventy-five percent of my time trying to persuade people that this approach always provides benefit and often abolishes symptoms completely.

Everyone is different so no two persons react to anything in exactly the same way. This kind of symptom complex is, however, extremely common. There are thousands, perhaps millions, of people whose daily lives are made miserable and have no idea why they feel this way. *Attention Deficit Disorder* (ADD) is increasingly common in children suffering from high calorie malnutrition. Sometimes a mother, consulting for her own health, will bring her child since she now recognizes the dietary association.

I particularly remember a fifteen-year-old girl. Every explanation offered was blocked by an angry emotional reaction that was irrational and communication was impossible. She had been brought for consultation because of her irrational and semi-violent behavior. In a disciplinary confrontation she would hit her parents and use foul language. Her diet was appalling and there was no hope of persuading her to change because there was no cognitive awareness. The primitive person who resides in all of us was "in charge" in this case.

If this is common enough, it is important to our culture and, indeed, our civilization. This fifteen-year-old girl had absolutely no concept that she was abnormal in her reactions. Could similar reactions be responsible for the disaster of Columbine? I have never seen any suggestion in any of the school shooting disasters that diet has been examined. The hedonistic diet to which our children have become accustomed is a logical precursor to the craving that might move from chocolate and sweets to the street drug scene. The mechanism of addiction is the same for

A Nutritional Approach to a Revised Model for Medicine

all addictive substances. It is merely an over-stimulation of the centers in the brain which deal with the sensation of pleasure. The more we stimulate these centers, the more we seek the stimulant. This leads to craving and it becomes the dominating preoccupation of the senses. It is only the degree of severity that separates the various common addictive substances. It is not easy for anyone to accept that a spectrum of apparently innocuous substances that give pleasure may not be so innocuous for some people. I recently was asked by an alcoholic whether I could help him. It is well known that alcoholism is associated with Vitamin B1 metabolism and I provided him with a disulfide derivative of thiamin that enables it to enter cells more easily than the Vitamin B1 sold at the health food store. His craving for alcohol was broken almost immediately and his health began to improve.

We are constantly adapting to our environment. For example we sweat when it is hot and shiver when it is cold. They are compensatory mechanism mediated through the autonomic nervous system which is controlled automatically by the computer where the changes are sensed. If these reactions are distorted we may experience a feeling of being hot or cold inappropriately in response to these environmental changes. As the Chinese philosophers stated, you do not want to be in a yang or a yin state permanently. You need to be at the point of balance between the two. An extreme position such as shivering or sweating is a temporary imbalance that is adaptive in nature.

Although these reflex actions are complex, they are really no different from the one that happens when a hand is placed on a hot stove. The hand is removed reflexly to reduce damage as much as possible and the pain comes a moment later. It is a protective reflex. In a sense we exist as two personalities. The lower brain presides over our primitive instinctive drives while the upper one acts as an advisor. When the dialogue between them is proceeding normally, we have sanity. The limbic brain is capable of doing something without the cognitive brain being consciously aware as in sleep walking. It is possible that it "takes over" under extreme provocation. The cognitive brain might be aware of the action, but powerless to stop it.

Since our primitive sex drive arises from the limbic computer, perhaps the "irrational" conduct of President Clinton was because of temporary over-ride of the limbic brain resulting in loss of the normal dialogue of inhibition. Perhaps this might have been related to his well advertised junk food ingestion. Limbic system provocations of this nature are more likely to occur and the craving for any addictive substance is increased under mental stress.

The problem of understanding a violent reaction under extreme emotional stress is that it is driven by a biochemical reaction of the computer. It is the limbic system that gives rise to the sensation of rage, and it is this system that will automatically send out instructions to the body through the nervous and endocrine systems. The facial appearance, the aggressive stance, the dilatation of the pupils, the pallor, the sweat that breaks out on the forehead, and the final reaction may all be perpetrated by the limbic system before it is perceived and modified by the conscious brain. This more easily happens when the limbic system has been changed biochemically and electrically. It is also important to add that the limbic brain can exert super-human strength when it reacts in this manner, explaining heroism as well as an act of violence, both of which are extraordinary.

The difference between a civilized person and a savage is that of programming by experience and teaching. But the machinery for savagery is just beneath the surface of all of us. If the "cave man within" is provoked enough by unusual circumstances, it becomes the "personality" that controls the action. One of the easiest ways to do this is through high calorie malnutrition, because these complex reflex reactions can be initiated with a trivial stimulus. This is particularly true in children. It is difficult, however, to persuade someone to discontinue "junk" items that give so much potentially addictive pleasure. Discontinuing them and taking a few nutritional supplements results in gradual change in personality and disappearance of the somatic symptoms. Perhaps we can explain the effects of alcohol as representing a form of acute high calorie malnutrition that overwhelms the ability of the enzymatic machinery to process it, thus explaining its well known association with Vitamin B1 deficiency, We must conclude that it is the ratio of calories to the vitamin/mineral nutrients required to process the calories like the analogy of the choked internal combustion engine.

CHAPTER 4

THE ROLE OF ENERGY METABOLISM

Newton examined the world and the heavens in visible terms. We were, however, unaware of the molecular components of matter until the modern era of physics, ushered in by Einstein and others. Einstein showed that matter and energy are interchangeable, and although it became the blueprint for the atomic bomb, it also led to an increased understanding of biological mechanisms.

The human body consists of seventy to one hundred trillion cells. Like citizens in an enormous and complex city, each must be regarded as an organism that has undergone evolutionary changes, endowing it with a special function. They form body organs like communities within a city. Relatively primitive as man is, he certainly has the capacity to appreciate the wonders of creation, but he has a long way to go in order to reach perfection. How can trillions of cells work together in a cooperative manner? It should be no surprise that the limbic system brain governs the body as a sophisticated computer. The brain/body relationship relies on communication depending on chemistry and electricity.

Energy Production

The body is a self-repairing machine that requires adequate energy for this task. Energy is produced in each of our cells by the process of oxidation, a sophisticated form of combustion. It involves combination of oxygen with fuel, requiring the presence of catalysts. We have many words in the English language for

A Nutritional Approach to a Revised Model for Medicine

combustion, the difference between them representing the speed of the reaction. A catalyst provides energy to ignite the fuel. Energy is always expended to create more energy and some is always lost in the transduction process. An internal combustion engine burns gasoline, but about sixty to seventy percent of the energy that is produced is lost in the form of noise, friction, and heat. It is therefore said to be about thirty to forty percent efficient. The human body is about seventy-five percent efficient.

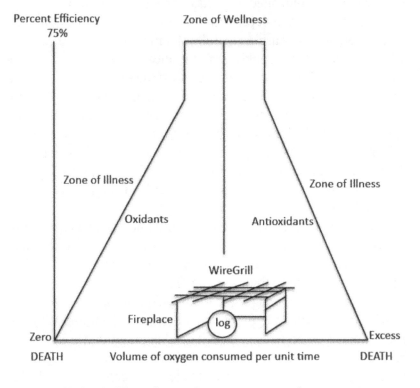

FIGURE 2: The volume of oxygen consumed per unit time

Figure 2 is a graph which shows oxygen use, on the horizontal axis, plotted against efficiency on the vertical axis. Efficiency is defined as the percentage of useful work performed in relation to the fuel consumed. The horizontal axis indicates the increasing amount of oxygen used (oxidation) as cells work harder in response to required mental or physical activity. Complete deprivation of oxygen is lethal, so efficiency will be zero on the left of the horizontal axis. Oxygen is also lethal in excess on the right hand end of the graph. Oxygen, the primary nutrient, is the decisive mechanism of healthy cellular energy metabolism. High pressure oxygen (hyperbaric oxygen) is sometimes used for treating some diseases but Figure 2 demonstrates that it has to be carefully controlled, or it has a potential for harm.

Although oxygen deprivation is lethal, oxygen "poisoning," is less well known. Turning to a simpler model, imagine a camper who wishes to start a cooking fire in a clearing in a forest (Figure 2). Since it risks setting fire to the forest, he takes the precaution of building a fireplace, thus controlling the fire. As it increases in intensity, more heat energy results and it may begin to throw out sparks that also might result in setting fire to the forest. A wire grill placed over the fire serves to catch and quench the sparks. The wire grill is composed of a number of wires, each of which is a cooperative member of the whole grill. A single wire would not do the job.

Each cell in the body has exactly the same logistical problems to solve. Calorie bearing food in the form of protein, fat, and carbohydrate has to be oxidized with maximum efficiency. We breathe in order to extract oxygen from the air. Breathing pure oxygen would be damaging if we breathed it all the time. That is why it is dosed in hyperbaric oxygen treatment and why air rather than oxygen is used in SCUBA. Hemoglobin enables the red blood cells to pick up molecules of oxygen and convey them to the tissues where they are unloaded and combined with the fuel in the process of oxidation.

When gasoline is burned in the cylinder of a car engine, it is the spark plug that causes ignition. In our body cells, we have vital chemical substances that fulfill the same role. Vitamins, so-called because they are vital to life, and minerals, both derived from our diet, catalyze oxidation. In chapter 3, we saw how the body machinery has to respond to stress, the daily challenges of existence. Just like a car that has to meet the stress of climbing a hill, so our body cells are signaled by the computer to increase their activity in order to mobilize the adaptive mechanisms by which we meet stress. Thus, the "fire" has to burn faster and there is an automatic increase in use of oxygen. This is represented in Figure 2 by the sloping line from the left to the rectangular area in the center. The vitamins that enable this to happen are called oxidants, the equivalent of spark plugs. Deficiency of oxidants is a cause of diseases like beriberi and pellagra, considered to be extinct in a modern developed society.

On the right side of Figure 2, oxygen is being lost from the reaction in the form of free oxygen radicals, the equivalent of sparks. Like sparks from a fire, they are thrown out when the oxidation mechanism becomes increasingly active to meet the demands of the stress. Just like the analogy of the fire, they are derived from a perfectly normal process of oxidation. Like sparks, however, they have to be quenched as they form and are therefore kept under control. This function is performed by a series of chemical substances called antioxidants.

Like the wire grill that is made up of separate units of wire which, together work as a team, antioxidants also work together. None of them have value alone since only collectively are they able to quench the "sparks." Some of the antioxidants, like Vitamins C and E are obtained from diet, but this is such a vital process that many of them are synthesized in the body. A study performed some years ago using beta carotene alone in treatment of disease, was predictably futile. Carotene is used in the body to produce Vitamin A and works only in conjunction with all the other non-caloric nutrients. Protection from "fire" is just as vital in the body as it is in a house or other building. Oxygen, used improperly in the complex processes of oxidation, is dangerous, and even lethal. It is another example of yin and yang. As we become older, it becomes more difficult for the body to produce those antioxidants that are normally synthesized in the body throughout life. They then have to be supplemented from diet. These, like coenzyme Q 10, are then known as conditional nutrients.

Oxidants and antioxidants have to be balanced. The rectangular area in Figure 2 represents the zone of maximum efficiency and oxygen consumption increases in proportion to the amount of work being performed. Under ideal conditions maximum efficiency is maintained at all times. The brain uses twenty-two and one-half times more oxygen per gram than that used by an equivalent mass of muscle at rest and is the reason why mental fatigue is more severe than that derived from purely physical means. The zone of illness is on either side of the central rectangular area that represents the zone of wellness and maximum efficiency. What cannot be predicted is the degree of inefficiency that will result in symptoms.

Loss of efficiency, represented on both sides of Figure 2, can occur at the same time because the oxidants are the "spark plugs" and the antioxidants the "firewall." An analogy for this balanced relationship might be the "cathedral roof" of nutrition or Yin and Yang, oxidants on the left and antioxidants on the right. The "roof" can be damaged by weakness or absence of one or more components. The task of nutritionists is to determine which of the many components may be missing, leading to loss of biochemical efficiency.

Simplicity must be derived out of complexity to be useful. Einstein probably used thousands of pages in working out the theory of relativity. The final equation, $E = mc^2$, can be understood in principle, since it tells us that matter and energy are convertible. Nomenclature of the huge number of described diseases has become complex because of the concept that each is a separate entity for which a specific cure must be found. The energy requiring mechanisms that the body uses to heal itself can only be supported through proper cellular fuel. Knowledge of how they are used is the essential factor. Drugs do nothing for the cause of the disease. They only treat symptoms.

Energy Synthesis

The energy storage compound that is used by all our cells is an unstable substance known as *adenosine triphosphate* (ATP). This is the energy storage equivalent of rolling a stone up a hill. The energy expended gives a stone potential energy that, in turn, can be expended by allowing it to roll down the hill. The rolling stone is a simple "engine," changing potential energy to kinetic energy. The formation of ATP in cells, although the details are widely different, can be compared with rolling the stone up a hill to form potential energy. It can be thought of as an "electronic hill."

Our cells are always "rolling a stone up an electronic hill and rolling it down the hill at the same time." It takes energy to make ATP and that has to be obtained from the fuel burning process (oxidation). Because ATP is being used and made at the same rate, the energy supply is maintained in a stable fashion. When we require more energy, ATP production is accelerated automatically in order to keep up with the increased workload.

Oxidative Metabolism

The primary fuel in animal biology is glucose, but we never find any form of sugar totally free in nature. It is always wrapped up in a fruit, a stem, a leaf, or a root. It is thus surrounded by fiber, a vital part of nutrition. All simple sugars are metabolized as glucose and absorbed from the bowel into the blood stream. The absorption is modified by the presence of fiber so that the reaction is slowed down, giving the brain/body mechanisms a chance to process the glucose. If it is taken as pure sugar, it stimulates the taste buds on the tongue and sends a message into the computer that is highly sensitive to a sudden increase in blood sugar. The computer over-reacts to the message input, inducing a message that results in secretion of insulin from the pancreas. It is therefore acting as a drug when used this way. It is the taste signal to the brain that is potentially addictive.

Glucose metabolism is a very complex series of biochemical reactions that convert it to *pyruvic* acid. This is fed into cellular machinery known as the citric acid cycle. Pyruvic acid is converted to another chemical and then it begins a chain of similar conversions that eventually return it to the beginning of the cycle, meanwhile giving off electrons in the form of energy. Each chemical reaction is governed by a genetically determined enzyme, each of which requires one or more vitamins and minerals to catalyze it. A simple Newtonian analogy is a crank-case in a car engine. An explosion in a cylinder moves a piston that drives the crank-case. The energy produced is transduced to kinetic energy through a transmission.

The citric acid cycle is the equivalent of the crank-case, involving electrical and chemical principles that occur in nearly every one of the seventy to one-hundred trillion cells that make up the body. As this biochemical "wheel" turns, it manufactures electrons that are picked up by a chemical substance called an electron carrier and delivered to a kind of electronic pipe-line known as the electron transfer chain. Without going into details, this synthesizes ATP and heat. The heat that is generated makes us warm-blooded creatures.

Generation of ATP might be compared with storage of electricity in a battery. Moving down an "electronic hill," it is converted to its lower energy form, *adenosine diphosphate* (ADP) and then to *adenosine monophosphate* (AMP) and finally to *adenosine*, three grades of energy loss similar to that which happens in a battery as the charge is lost in performing work. The loss of each phosphate molecule in this manner can be compared with the Newtonian equivalent of a stone rolling down a hill. Adenosine is continuously built up again by adding phosphate molecules to synthesize ATP, similar to recharging a battery. This is a continuous process of energy formation and usage and the two must always be balanced. As this energy transduction takes place, water as the final oxidation product, is formed. If the electrons pass through the chain and fail to

A Nutritional Approach to a Revised Model for Medicine

"charge the ATP battery" the expenditure of energy is useless in life cell maintenance and only heat energy is formed. This is what happens, for example, when too much thyroid hormone circulates because, in excess, this hormone creates adverse changes in the electron transfer chain.

All of this complex machinery is housed in the cell membrane that surrounds the *mitochondria*. They represent the "fireplaces" and are the "micro-machines" where oxidation takes place to manufacture ATP. They also require "fire protection" as already described. A membrane encloses each of our body cells, and a similar membrane encloses the mitochondria. Each membrane is like a two-walled house, and the electron transfer machinery is in the inner half of the membrane. Making these discoveries is a remarkable feat in itself, enabling us to incorporate the knowledge into a new perspective of health and disease.

The thyroid gland might be compared with an engine that is equipped with a fly-wheel. The hormone it produces allows metabolism to increase or decrease in speed, thus acting as a metabolic governor. *Hyperthyroidism,* also known as Grave's Disease, causes energy to be dissipated in the form of heat with insufficient ATP synthesis. Before the action of the thyroid gland was better understood, doctors were confronted sometimes with a patient suffering a "thyroid storm," a lethal condition caused by insufficiency of ATP while heat energy was being formed in excess.

Many years ago it was discovered that a drug called *dinitrophenylhydrazine* (DNP) caused people to lose weight. Some consumers suddenly died because DNP interferes with the normal process of energy transduction just described. DNP is now used on experimental animals in researching energy metabolism. This drug has recently been advertized again on-line and is extremely dangerous, thus accentuating the lack of adequate control over information available on the Internet. Commercial drive, though a necessary component of modern life, becomes a severe threat when used in a state of ignorance or, worse yet, when the money becomes more important than life itself. This illustrates the problem of drug safety and we still keep coming upon examples of dangerous side effects from drugs. Drug reactions are quite common and seem to be accepted as part of the risk of treating disease. If people took the trouble to read the *Physicians' Desk Reference* about their medications, many would refuse to take them.

Sometimes the Treatment Is More Dangerous Than the Disease

The human body is a self-repairing machine dependent upon a supply of energy to each of our body cells. Thinking is brain work that requires energy. Because it is silent and not associated with any observable physical movement we do not always realize that we are consuming fuel at a greater rate than muscles that carry out purely physical work. Thus, energy consumption is greater in mental rather than physical work, explaining why mental fatigue is a different sensation from that experienced from physical work. This is the reason why our brightest children are at greatest risk from bad diet. Hyperactive and inattentive grade school students are almost always described as "bright" by parents. Reports by teachers often indicate that such a child (most often a boy) is not reaching his potential and it is difficult for some parents to grasp the fact that their "erring child" is a biochemical rather than a psychological problem. I must emphasize again that the limbic system brain computer becomes irritable when energy metabolism within it is inefficient, and this is giving rise to so much illness that is classified as "psychological, mental, or psychiatric" in nature.

The energy produced in the engine of a car has to be transmitted to the driving wheels by means of a transmission. The energy produced in cells has to be used to provide function so there has to be the equivalent of a transmission, another complex biochemical process that consumes energy. It has been shown, for example, that the "transmission" is defective in children with autism. The automatic brain conducts the adaptive mechanisms of the body by means of various forms of communication, the endocrine, and autonomic nervous systems being the main means of conveying the messages. Both systems are controlled by the limbic system computer, enabling us to adapt to the constant changes that we meet in our environment. This might be thought of as the equivalent of a transmission.

The Role of Calcium

When a body cell receives a signal from the computer, calcium ions pass into the cell and cause it to become active. Part of the ensuing activity of the cell is to pump out the calcium, allowing it to go back to a resting state. It then awaits another signal before it works again. In an organ made up of millions of similar cells, all programmed to perform their individual tasks, they are not all working at the same time. Some are working while others are resting and that means that each cell has an opportunity to rebuild its product and its energy stores ready for the next challenge issued from the message center.

Body cells have to be healthy for this complex and repetitive mechanism to continue smoothly throughout their limited lifetime. In a state of optimum health our body cells are being destroyed and replaced by new ones throughout life. One of the mechanisms causing one form of heart attack is a massive influx of calcium into cells within the walls of arteries that feed the heart, causing them to constrict. A stress event, such as reading a telegram that brings bad news, causes the corresponding emotion, derived from a series of automatic signals in the computer. Physical stress, such as shoveling snow, also results in adaptive signals from the computer to organize the necessary increase in energy. Either emotional or physical stress sends a signal through the autonomic nervous system that accelerates the heart. If cells receiving the signals are unhealthy, or if the signals received are in a massive volume, the influx of calcium can cause arterial constriction that results in heart attack. It is the computerized reaction that different forms of stress initiates that is lethal and that depends upon the health of the individual as a whole. Any stress input is data processed by the brain computer that then automatically tells the body how to adapt. A failure in this dynamic mechanism results in a maladaptive response that might be lethal. The health of cell membranes is crucial to the reception of signals as well as the ability of the cell to absorb nutrients, including oxygen. Cell membranes are semi-fluid, a little like soap bubbles, and one of the most important aspects of research is how this state of fluidity is maintained. It is one of the obvious reasons why diet is so crucial to health. Millions of molecules, discovered, named, and reported in medical literature are really chemical messengers. They make up the "language" of communication between all our cells. They are really the "gophers" of the coordination mechanism, like pageboys in a large organization.

Mitochondria

Mitochondria are the engines of the cell. If they are unable to produce sufficient "horsepower" for the activities of cells, the affected cells will not function properly. Each of our cells is governed by genes that are provided by both parents and carry our genetically determined characteristics. But the mitochondria have their own genes that are passed only from the mother. Mitochondrial DNA is circular rather than linear as it is in cellular genes, one of the characteristics of bacterial DNA. The evidence is that mitochondria evolved from an ancient bacterium that infected a cell millions of years ago. It is as though the bacterium evolved in a symbiotic manner in return for "room and board." The mitochondrial genes from the father are carried in the tail of the sperm and are lost in the act of fertilization of the ovum, thus leaving the maternal mitochondrial genes as the inherited link. Mitochondrial DNA mutates much more often than nuclear DNA, producing one form of a maternally derived genetically determined disease. It has been found that the reduced energy power of affected cells can sometimes be improved by supplementing nutrition with specific vitamins and minerals.

This form of inheritance produces serious functional ability and is relatively uncommon. If the mother's health problems are caused this way, she can pass the defect to all of her children. The commonest way to cause the symptoms of energy deficiency, however, is through bad diet, particularly simple sweet carbohydrate. It is the easiest way to cause stress to be converted into disease. Because the limbic brain is so energy demanding, the control of the autonomic nervous system becomes unbalanced and its exaggerated function gives rise to symptoms that may be emotional or somatic in nature or both together. Thus, a change in barometric pressure or environmental temperature, acting as sensory input to the computer, might result in symptoms arising from exaggerated activity of autonomic signals. The "stressor," in this example, is a natural phenomenon to which we have to adapt. If the normal adaptive machinery is distorted by this means, the patient is maladapted to the environment. He/she may complain, for example, of being hot when in a cool ambient temperature, or vice versa. Other symptoms arising from breakdown of autonomic control result in the syndrome of functional *dysautonomia*. Although this condition will not be found in a textbook, it is quite often reported in the medical literature associated with a number of diseases. These reports are published to note that autonomic dysfunction has been found to relate to a specific disease such as lung cancer. In none of the publications has there been an attempt to explain the association. There is evidence, however, that both aspects of this association can be related to loss of efficiency in oxidative metabolism in the body as a whole.

Since mitochondrial disease can be acquired, it is the major cause of *Chronic Fatigue Syndrome* (CFS) generally considered to be related to viral infection with, for example, the Epstein

Barr virus, the cause of mononucleosis. CFS often starts with a flu-like illness, often treated unwisely with antibiotics. As symptoms such as fatigue and muscle pain develop and become chronic, the treatment is the initiating mechanism. Antibiotics are designed to kill bacteria. If mitochondria have a structure in their DNA that is similar to that found in bacteria, it might be logical to ask whether the widespread use of these drugs might be responsible for a large number of cases of CFS by damaging cellular mitochondria. Perhaps the drugs only knock out a percentage of them in a number of body cells and we know that some mitochondria can be disabled while others are working normally. The fact is that each cell has a large number of mitochondria, and when it divides to make new cells, they have to be passed into the daughter cells. If only a percentage of the mitochondria are dysfunctional and the remainder normal, the energy generated will be proportional. The latest science of epigenetics has shown that DNA can, in fact, be changed chemically by poor diet and lifestyle

When someone sees a physician today with a cold, "flu," or any other viral infection, he can expect to have an antibiotic prescribed. This is in the face of common knowledge that these drugs do not affect viruses. If the physician is asked why he is prescribing such a drug, he will often reply that it is "to take care of the possible secondary invasion of bacteria." While this may be a legitimate concern, it may only complicate the situation. Unfortunately medico-legal risk enters the equation. The history of CFS is so repetitive that it is almost guaranteed that antibiotics have been prescribed, sometimes for years, even as the symptoms have become more and more chronic. Nutrients, the only way to treat CFS, may have to be given intravenously because the bowel cells of many such people are also energy damaged and this may result in malabsorption of nutrients. I call the treatment mitochondrial resuscitation rather than cure, emphasizing that nutrients support energy requiring natural healing. If and when the mitochondria become more efficient, the symptoms begin to fall away and a percentage of former health returns. The response is variable, but at the very least it does no harm, thus obeying the Hippocratic Oath. If any treatment is more harmful than the disease, it should not be used. Unfortunately we have been "brainwashed" by the pharmaceutical industry. We have to take a brand new look at what we are doing and Alternative Medicine is doing just that. It is seeking methods to assist the healing process.

The present method of classifying disease is in keeping with the model as it now exists. This is because of the concept that each disease is a separate process generated by a definitive cause, "the enemy." We are surrounded with microorganisms that are our only predators, conforming with Darwin's philosophy, survival of the fittest. Opportunist microorganisms, waiting for physiological body deterioration, seize their opportunity and become activated. As Louis Pasteur said on his death bed, "I was wrong (about attacking microorganisms). It is the terrain (body defenses) that matters." A basic understanding of the brain/body function and the role of energy is vital in maintaining our own health. The 21st century should see an enormous change in the way that we deal with health problems. The word "doctor" must be returned to its original meaning of "teacher" and the advice given to patients will depend upon their sufficient understanding of their own responsibilities and the choices that they make in nutrition and lifestyle. We use the word "energy" to describe physical function when we say that someone is extremely active. What we forget is the fact that such activity is consuming cellular energy. Thus, many people are using caffeine in order to "get to work" because they are so fatigued and do not seem to have benefitted from a night's sleep. What they are failing to recognize is that they are simply stimulating cellular function that consumes energy that they can ill afford. The underlying mechanism of their fatigue is lack of efficiency in the mitochondria, the "engines" of the cell. By far and away the commonest cause is poor diet as I have repeatedly emphasized in these pages.

CHAPTER 5

A REVISED MEDICAL MODEL

The change from health to disease requires a model. It should be clear that the brain and body work as parts of the same "machine" and this would seem to be so obvious that it does not require stating. The present medical model, however, regards them as separate entities. Hence we talk of mental disease in a different category from physical disease. If dysfunction of the body arises as a result of brain action it is called psychosomatic. The brain and body are in a constant state of dialogue, most of which goes on below conscious awareness. The lower brain is clearly a computer since it acts automatically and does not require volition. The nervous system that innervates the bowel is so complex that it has been thought of as the second brain. For every signal to the bowel from the brain there are as many as nine signals from the bowel to the brain. The limbic system "talks" to the cognitive brain and to the organs of the body by means of messengers and the body "talks" back to the brain. The model described here differs from the one that is presently used in our explanation of disease. Hundreds of different diseases have been described, based on constellations of symptoms and clinical observations derived from physical examination of the patient. The names given to them are descriptive in nature and provide little or no information about their underlying cause. A physician then has to consider what is termed a "differential diagnosis," memorizing those diseases that might or might not fit the description by the patient and what the physician finds on physical examination.

A Nutritional Approach to a Revised Model for Medicine

Laboratory tests are used to support or rule out the diagnostic category proposed. If the tests for a given disease are positive, the diagnosis is confirmed. If they are negative, the physician must look further. The goal is to identify the disease accurately so that the most modern drug treatment available might be used. If there are no abnormalities in the physical examination and the laboratory tests are all normal, the patient is considered to have no "organic" disease and the condition is often then termed "functional" or "psychosomatic," a term that suggests the problem to be "psychological." By this, it is meant to suggest that the patient is nervous or is a hypochondriac, implying that the nervousness is responsible for the symptoms.

This approach has a kind of "hit-or-miss" quality that is disturbing. Because of the infinite number of permutations and combinations of ways in which the body generates symptoms, we have written millions of pages in books that document the variations in disease expression. There are "new" diseases that occasionally appear and the unfortunate medical student is supposed to memorize them. One particularly nasty way in which this is imposed upon the student is by the use of "syndromes." A syndrome is a collection of symptoms, signs and laboratory data (if laboratory work has been identified in association with the syndrome) that were first described by a physician. The disease entity is then known as "John Doe's Syndrome" and the name of the describer goes down in medical history. If that particular constellation of facts is observed in a given patient, it is written in the medical records as a syndrome with the name of the original describer attached. The point is that it adds absolutely nothing to our knowledge of the cause of that constellation of symptoms. In addition, a physician is regarded as being ignorant if the mention of the syndrome is not recognized. Presumably, he/she is expected to remember all these syndromes in understanding the patient's problems of health disorder.

If the diagnosis is considered to be "functional," or "psychosomatic", meaning that there is no organic disease present to explain the symptoms, a psychologist or psychiatrist will explore the patient's background according to the teaching of Freud or one of his disciples. A psychiatrist may prescribe the latest drug that suppresses symptoms but does not address the underlying biochemical relationship with symptoms. The term "functional" came into common use because it is considered that functions have become deviant but that there is no evidence for an underlying physical disease. The idea of there being abnormal biochemistry is relatively new and very few physicians accept that malnutrition could be related. Dr. Linus Pauling wrote a paper in *Science* in 1971 that gave us the word "orthomolecular." This simply means that any cell in the body requires the complement of essential nutrients that enable it to function efficiently.

It seems that patients have come to accept the orthomolecular concept more readily than their physicians. They want to know if they are out of balance in a chemical sense. If the symptoms are clearly arising because of devious activity in the computer, they have almost always been treated as exhibiting "psychological" abnormality and either counseling or a drug has been used to attempt treatment. In fact, the very word "treatment" implies that the doctor is in charge of the situation and is regarded as "the healer." On many occasions, the side effects from drugs have been worse than the original condition. It is therefore not really surprising that many people are seeking other methods of identifying their problems, even in spite of the present lack of insurance coverage for the various methods used in the broadening field of what has come to be known as Complementary Alternative Medicine (CAM). Using the term complementary (often confused with complimentary) indicates that organized mainline medicine has indeed come a long way, but needs to be complemented by a number of techniques and treatments that are not based on pharmaceutical drugs.

In order to understand the nature of the symptoms, it is necessary to use the brain-body model already introduced.

A Nutritional Approach to a Revised Model for Medicine

We need to wipe out preconceived notions about the differences between psychological and physical and think of the fact that each of us has two brains. Of course we have only one brain from an anatomical point of view. As discussed in chapter 3, however, it must be thought of as being compartmentalized into the lower brain computer and the upper cognitive or conscious brain. The dialogue between them is necessary for a "civilized" or thoughtful person to emerge. I emphasize that again, because we do have a more primitive lower brain that is the "cave man" that lies within each one of us. We are all capable of mayhem and other less pleasant human activities. If the dialogue between the two is distorted, we begin to see the seeds of "madness."

The brains of higher animals in the animal kingdom are built on the same basic principle. The lowest part is the most primitive and is obviously a computer as already discussed. Layers have been added through evolution and each layer increases the sophistication. We believe that we have the most sophisticated brain in the animal kingdom, enabling us to perform very complex actions, but it is completely dependent upon a normal dialogue between its various components, each of which is specialized to perform its individual tasks. If the dialogue between the primitive limbic system and the cognitive or conscious brain breaks down, we may have one definition of "madness." It is unfortunate in this scientific age that the overwhelming evidence for evolution is being denied by many and "creationists" abound. They will have difficulty in accepting what is written here, since it depends on the fact that the human brain has indeed evolved and that we still have its most primitive components.

Everything that happens to us gives rise to an impulse in our nervous perception apparatus. This means, of course, that the input from all our senses is being continuously passed into the computer for data processing. Visual, auditory, olfactory, and tactile stimuli are perceived throughout a lifetime. When we are asleep, it is the auditory pathway that is most easily stimulated to awaken us, and that makes sense. It would be an act of survival to maintain an open hearing sense in the wild state. A Japanese soldier lived in the jungle for years after the end of World War II, because he did not know that it was over. It was reported that his hearing was so acute that he could hear his clothes rubbing against his skin when he moved. This particular sense had been honed to this degree of awareness by the process of adapting to the extreme potential hostility of his environment. This is probably the kind of sensory perception that we had when we were living in caves since it would have improved our chances of survival.

This sensory input is the way that we perceive our environment. Without the necessary interpretation imposed by the brain as it receives this information, we would not have any idea that our environment actually exists. For example, most of us believe that we taste with the tongue. What really happens is that the tongue senses the taste stimulus and is equipped to send a message to the brain where the signal is interpreted. We taste, detect odors, hear, see, and touch with our brains. The organs that transmit the signals have to communicate with the brain, or no perception is possible. We need to be careful to differentiate between the input and the data processing reaction in the computer. Stress is defined here to indicate only the causative change in the environment that results in stimulation. This causes "input" to the computer through the various senses that we possess. Input stimulation provides information to the computer where it is data processed, resulting in a chemical reaction that then has to be interpreted. A gentle stroking of the skin results in a sense of tranquility and peace. An insult results in the sensation of anger. A telegram that delivers bad news causes depression or grief. The computer is programmed to respond in the expected manner to the quality and interpretation of the stimulus.

Each emotion is accompanied by appropriate messages to the body which are essentially adaptive in nature. Depression, for example, is a normal chemical reaction to bad news. If it is initiated without a recognizable stimulus and is prolonged, it is still the same mechanism but abnormally exaggerated due to faulty chemistry. It is irrational because it is "without reason."

Adaptive Physical Reactions.

Many complex body reactions are automated. Sweating occurs when we go into a hot environment and shivering in a cold one. Both represent the opposite extremes of a normal reaction to environmental temperature. Both are "ordered" by the brain computer and are compensatory, the yin and the yang of our daily experiences. If the computer is deranged in a chemical sense, it may initiate sweating without any environmental necessity. In today's world of high stress and excessive coffee intake, this is extremely common. The message is delivered through the sympathetic branch of the autonomic system, the mechanism that guards us from harm by adapting us to that environment. An emotion is like a "file" in the "hard drive" that emerges with the proper stimulus. The computer becomes very much more reactive when its energy metabolism is inefficient and high calorie malnutrition is the easiest way to produce it. I have even compared its effects with those of lead poisoning that afflicted the ancient Romans. Although lead is a known poison and high calorie malnutrition would seem to be very far removed from that, it is not known by many that lead in infinitesimally small concentrations is a nutrient. A completely lead-free diet, an extremely difficult one to prepare, was given to animals that failed to grow until lead traces were restored. Until 1957 selenium was regarded as a poison, just like lead, but it is now known to be an essential nutrient. It is, however, required in extremely minute doses and is toxic in larger amounts. It is possible that we may require the entire periodic table of elements, thus making the formula used at the burial service "earth to earth and dust to dust" logical.

Allergy

In a routine case history, many people complain of allergies, no matter what the main complaint may be. This is so common that it has almost become acceptable as a normal part of life. The diagnosis is often made by an allergist by performing various tests. Medications or injections are commonly used for treatment with variable success. The usual symptoms are nasal congestion, watering eyes, and recurrent sinus problems, often called "hay fever" if it is seasonal. In a comprehensive questionnaire given to new patients, I have found that nasal congestion is extremely common, usually in the morning on awakening. In some cases the patient has been subjected to an operation to straighten the nasal septum, a procedure that I find hard to understand. Nasal sprays often make it gradually worse and antihistamines have their side effects. Food allergy affects people who cannot eat certain foods because they generate unpleasant symptoms. The explanation offered here depends on the previous chapters.

The computer is continuously notified concerning internal mechanisms in the body as well as of environmental change. When food goes into the stomach, it automatically signals the brain computer as shown in Figure 3.

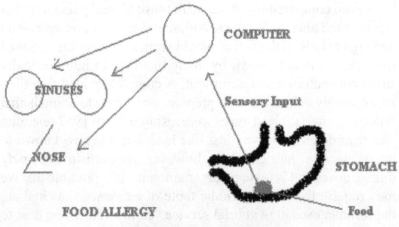

FIGURE 3: Food Allergy

A Nutritional Approach to a Revised Model for Medicine

As the stomach fills with food, the signals crescendo and it is the brain that determines a sense of fullness. In a healthy person this communication between the stomach and a satiety center in the hypothalamus results in an intake of food that is proportional to needs. Fat containing cells secrete a hormone called *leptin* that travels in the blood to the hypothalamus where it signals the excess of fat. Genetically obese mice become normally lean when injected with leptin and it looked like a good idea for obese humans. It was found that the hypothalamus in obese humans was resistant to the action of leptin, thus underscoring the fact that obesity is a much more complex problem than merely reducing caloric intake. We now know that the hypothalamus, the center of the "computer," plays an extremely important part in both obesity and inflammation. Thus, we have a potential explanation for widespread obesity and its now well known association with inflammatory disease.

It is the activity of the computer that causes the symptoms because it has been made more reactive to incoming signals. Common causes include chronic ingestion of coffee and various forms of "junk" diet. As shown in Figure 3, this may result in the computer sending out executive commands to the nose and the sinuses, signaling the cells in the mucous membrane within those organs to produce mucus. Mucus provides lubrication that maintains surface moisture, and is protective of the delicate tissues involved. If, however, the computer sends an overactive signal to those glands, they will react in the way that they are programmed and produce an excess of mucus. The sinuses have drainage holes in them that enable the mucus to be discharged into the nose. Pressure in the sinuses may give rise to headache but if bacteria get into a mucus filled sinus, it will find a good culture medium and cause sinusitis. The initial reaction is purely reflex and may be only a part of the maladaptive reaction that the computer generates. If the appropriate preventive action is taken, there never will be a "sinus infection." The best way is to cause the computer to become normally reactive instead of being hyper-responsive and firing out unnecessary executive signals. This is accomplished through proper nutrition.

Allergies of all sorts disappear in people when their nutrition is adequate to meet their energy needs. Food processing alters natural foods and may be the responsible factor in causing the allergic symptoms. For example, cows are given bovine growth hormone to increase milk production and antibiotics to prevent inflammation of the udder. Cow's milk was intended for calves until they can eat grass. It is hard to understand how cow's milk has become a health drink for humans. The milk of a mammal is intended as a temporary food for its young.

This explains why treatment of allergies requires supplemental vitamin/mineral nutrients. Ingestion of any offending food must be avoided until the computer has been restored to a state of normal efficiency.

An illustration of brain/body action is exemplified by the case of a woman who was known to be allergic to rose pollen. One day, she went into a room where there was a bowl of roses on the table. She developed asthma and had to be taken to hospital. It was then found that the roses were artificial. The important point is that the physical reflexes that were responsible for the asthma were induced by the purely visual observation of something to which the woman's brain computer had been programmed. It could not have been the physical effect of pollen in this case. Because the computer was programmed to react to rose pollen, the visual signal, through association with the control centers, was just as important as the tactile or molecular signal received from the nose when pollen alighted on its mucous membrane. Whenever I tell that story, my listener usually smiles since the reaction is thought to be somehow faked or "psychological," implying that it is the fault of the unfortunate individual in reacting this way.

Nasal congestion is extremely common, even in patients who are suffering from problems other than allergy. Since it is merely accepted by most people as normal, it is rarely volunteered. It is, however, revealed in a routine questionnaire that I ask every patient to fill in on the first consultation. One of the interesting phenomena is unilateral nasal congestion that occurs when a person is lying in bed trying to go to sleep. When he/she turns over, the nasal congestion clears in the originally affected nostril and reappears in the other. This is because sensory signals from the side of the body in contact with the bed go into the computer and initiate the executive signals to the nose. It is the overactive computer that is the cause. It also emphasizes the fact that the computer organizes adaptive signals in each half of the body separately. When the patient is lying on one side it results in input that causes asymmetric action to the mucus secreting gland of one nostril. When the patient turns over the signals go to the other nostril.

The same thing may happen when a particle of dust alights on the mucous membrane of the nose. A signal to the computer depends on the threshold of its executive action. It may simply result in sneezing, or a much wider reaction referred to as an allergy. If sensory cells in the local area, the nose, take care of the problem, that person would never know of the event. Under normal health conditions the computer does not overreact because it recognizes that there is no danger arising to the well being of the organism from this tiny amount of dust and no executive action is required by central control.

It might be that to stop this kind of allergic reaction would be to discontinue taking coffee! Certainly such advice stretches credibility, but I remember a woman whom I had advised in this manner. I saw her again about a month after she had withdrawn from taking only two cups of coffee a day. After she discontinued it, she experienced a headache that lasted for forty-eight hours. This was so severe that she had stayed in bed. The headache then ceased and her health began to improve immediately. One of her major complaints had been severe fatigue. Two cups of coffee a day would affect very few, illustrating that we are all different in our responses to the environment in which we live. The advice given to this patient would be thought by most people to be absurd and the advice to discontinue the coffee would be ignored.

Many people have to have a cup of coffee to overcome fatigue while driving to work. If they stop taking it they suffer withdrawal headache, one of the characteristics of addiction. If the drugs were cocaine or alcohol this would be expected. Discontinuation would be recognized as the way to escape the addiction. Sometimes a coffee addict may interpret disappearance of withdrawal headache by taking yet another cup of coffee as a sign that he needs it. The amount of coffee is expected to be proportional to its untoward effects, whereas it is the sensitivity of the brain that counts. Cutting back on intake is ineffective and often leads to increased severity of symptoms with a lower dose. Only "cold turkey" will work. Most people would believe that two cups of coffee a day could not possibly be the factor that is causing the health problem. We all know of people who drink far more than this and do not have symptoms arising from it. I do think that it was absurd for Dr. Weiss to write an article in *Time* magazine advising that everyone should be drinking seven or eight cups of coffee a day, based on its antioxidant content. The effect of the caffeine content frequently outweighs the antioxidant benefit.

It is the reaction that results from the repeated sensory stimulation of the computer that counts. Thus coffee, sugar, chocolate, and a variety of soft drinks, especially those containing caffeine, are being taken as drugs. They are not poisonous in the accepted meaning of that word. They provide us with sensory pleasure by stimulating specialized brain cells. Pleasure sensation is something that we all seek in a variety of ways and is not, of itself, wrong. Over-stimulation is hedonistic. Thus addiction to coffee or sugar, the two most common drugs in our society, may lead to more emotional irritability and over-response to stimulus. Often there is a combination of both mental and somatic response that might erroneously be called psychosomatic.

There are only two things that we need to do in order to maintain health, assuming that a genetic background is not the most responsible factor. The first is to remove the offending substance if that is possible. This may be in minute quantity. A bee sting that might in some people be lethal is caused by a minute injection of formic acid. The reaction is disproportionate to the quantity and reflects the sensitivity of the individual's computer rather than the guaranteed danger of the bee sting alone.

We are deluded into believing that virtually all our activities are willed when we are conscious and awake. The involuntary and voluntary systems are integrated. Because we are not consciously aware of automatic input signals to the computer, we are only aware of the resulting reactions. If they are exaggerated they produce symptoms.

Irritable Bowel Syndrome

Easily recognized by anyone who has experienced this troublesome affliction, there is a sudden need to visit the toilet where diarrhea may or may not be experienced. This may happen several times a day and is particularly common in the morning. The diarrhea may be explosive and fluid in character, often accompanied by mucus and is frequently signaled by abdominal pain. It is often preceded by noises from the abdomen which are sometimes referred to as "growling" or "hunger pains" called *borborygmi*. Most people with this syndrome have other symptoms caused by increased autonomic activity.

The bowel is frequently a victim of unnecessarily violent signals that arise from the computer, although it is sometimes also inflamed as part of the computerized reaction that will be discussed later in the chapter. Morning activity is because it is associated with the brain rhythm known as Circadian. Messages through the autonomic nervous system result in unusually violent peristalsis, the wave-like motions of the bowel that carry its contents down for eventual elimination. As this occurs normally, digestion takes place and the nutrient components are absorbed through the bowel wall and enter the blood stream to be conveyed to the liver where they are processed. At the same time, water is removed from the contents of the bowel and a formed stool is eventually delivered to the terminal bowel where it is stored until evacuation takes place.

Because the peristaltic wave is grossly exaggerated, there is insufficient time for the normal processes to take place. The semi-solid contents of the upper bowel, where the process of digestion is occurring, are squeezed violently causing the *borborygmi*. The exaggerated wave pattern causes colicky abdominal pain. The bowel has a very complicated nervous system as mentioned in a previous chapter and it has been called "the second brain." Because it is a "two-way street" the initiating mechanism for diarrhea may be in the bowel itself, but the involvement of the brain computer is often solely responsible.

Most of the usual treatments are drugs that cut down the violence of the peristaltic waves but the patient is seldom asked about the important "drugs" that are taken daily. Common causes include coffee, chocolate, fruit juice, sugar, candy, etc. This is why a person with this syndrome almost always has other, usually unmentioned, symptoms derived from the irritable computer and revealed only by seeking a detailed history of the patient's overall health. It is usually regarded as a problem for a gastro-enterologist, but the patient is not suffering from an unhealthy bowel in an otherwise healthy body. The fault lies in the overactive messaging between the brain computer and bowel.

If there is an additional concomitant complaint of nasal congestion due to allergy, the presently used model of disease would consider the patient to have two diseases. If there was some anxiety or depression associated with these physical symptoms, the collection of symptoms might be called psychosomatic. A common way in which this may be handled is for a different specialist to be required for each complaint, since each one is considered to be outside the experience of the other consulted specialists.

School Phobia

A child, usually a boy, goes to school. On arrival, he complains of abdominal pain or headache and may even vomit. He is taken to the school nurse who calls his mother who takes him home. When he gets home, these symptoms disappear and he appears to be quite normal in every way. This scenario is repeated and it is not surprising that it is interpreted as a psychological problem. Such a child is usually referred to a psychologist.

The reality is that the child's limbic system has been set up in the same way as described above for irritable bowel syndrome, the commonest cause being bad diet. It has become "stress prone" which means that it overreacts to virtually any form of stress input, whether it be physical or mental. Going to school is an inevitable form of mental "stress." It is what all children experience going to school, but the reaction to it is increased and becomes "physical" in the phobic child. It is a maladaptive reaction. The stress (of going to school) causes exaggerated autonomic nervous system activity, resulting in the symptoms. Vomiting, if it occurs, is because the vomiting center in the brain stem is over-stimulated. It is an action of this center that induces vomiting, not the stomach.

A child with this condition is only functionally abnormal. It is only essential to stop providing him with the "junk" that is causing irritability in his limbic system. These children are usually quite bright. They like school and they usually like the teacher. They also may initially have plenty of friends. The irony of the situation is that a high-grade intelligence requires ideal nutrition. You cannot put bad fuel into a well built machine! The inappropriate label of psychological disease acts as a stress itself and may eventually result in additional personality changes, including withdrawal from other children.

Derrick Lonsdale M.D.

Pre Menstrual Syndrome

This affliction is affecting as many as thirty million young American women! It is not a gynecological disease. It is yet another disorder of the brain limbic system that controls the actions of glands in the endocrine system. These glands release the various hormones that circulate in the blood and are controlled by a biofeedback loop system between the affected organs and the brain computer. It is the limbic system that is in charge of the menstrual cycle and there are millions of messages that have to go back and forth between the body and the brain in order to organize it.

In the week before menstruation occurs, the messages are escalating as the preparations are made each month to enable the acceptance in the uterus of a fertile egg. Biochemical changes in the brain are responsible. Since it is responsible for our emotional reactions it is not surprising that emotional lability is part of the syndrome. Appetite controls are also in the limbic brain so there may be either loss of this or unusual hunger. Chocolate and/or salt craving are frequently experienced at this time because of the stimulation of the cells that control this mechanism. It has nothing to do with traditional psychology as the cause, although it certainly may become secondarily involved, particularly if conventional treatment is ineffective. The birth control pill, often used to treat the condition, may make the symptoms worse.

Knowledge about the brain/body model makes this syndrome easy to understand. But in the age of medical specialization, the patient may be referred to other physicians for a variety of symptoms.

For example, if the patient complains of palpitations of the heart, she may be sent to a cardiologist. If the cardiologist finds mitral valve prolapse, a condition affecting one of the heart valves in six to ten percent of the population, it then becomes the focus of attention. This is irrespective of the fact that this condition is usually, if not invariably, associated with disorganization of the autonomic nervous system, probably the real underlying cause.

If she is nervous or has mood swings, depression or panic attacks, she is referred to a psychologist or psychiatrist, and usually winds up with a drug that is unnecessary except, perhaps as a temporary symptomatic therapy.

If she has diarrhea, she is referred to a gastro-enterologist who treats the bowel, although this is not the real seat of the problem. The bowel is the victim of the computer signals described above. All of these symptoms are caused by an overactive computer. If this part of the brain is disturbed, everything else will be affected.

Although the birth control pill is used to treat gynecological disorders, it plays a large part in causing PMS in some women. The brain controls the complex hormonal balance in this monthly cycle and because of the biofeedback loop the administration of the hormones has an effect on it. This disorganization begins to affect the autonomic nervous system and this causes a lot of the symptoms. Many women discontinue use of the pill because of associated emotional lability, fatigue, bloating, and water retention. These obvious side effects are because of the abnormal dialogue that exists between the body organs and the controlling limbic system computer.

Circadian Rhythm

The word Circadian means "about twenty-four hours." Within the brain we have a biologic clock. It obeys the light/dark cycle in our twenty-four hour world and in women there is a normal cycle of twenty-eight days as well. That, after all, is why it is called "the period." We do not know whether men have a twenty-eight day cycle, because there is nothing to show for it. It would be surprising, however, if there was not such a cycle in men. It may well be that it is actually related to recurrent symptoms that are never thought of as being periodic. In the agricultural culture that we used to live in, our physiology meshed with Circadian rhythm. We went to bed when it became dark and arose with the sun. In the artificial, commercially driven world of today, we take little notice of these rhythmic pulses. They are, however still very important and some disease is associated with ignoring them. At about four o'clock in the afternoon, the computer begins to shut down our metabolic processes, presumably for energy conservation. At four in the morning it begins to revive our metabolism ready for the day's activity. That means that we are always adapting in the northern and southern hemispheres because of the seasonal changes in the dark/light cycle. It is also interesting that we now know that the natural Circadian rhythm is actually a twenty-five-hour cycle, suggesting the possibility that we are provided with a rhythm that has to be contracted to a twenty-four-hour world. We are thus forced to adapt to the constant changes in environment that we encounter throughout life, an unconscious process that is governed automatically in a healthy person. Nerves run from the retina in the eye back to a gland at the back of the brain known as the pineal. This secretes the hormone melatonin and one of its functions is to prepare us for sleep. Thus it is a dark sensitive mechanism and is the reason that we are ready for sleep at night under normal healthy conditions.

It is well known that some people become more depressed in the winter, the so-called "winter blues." If this becomes exaggerated in intensity, it can become pathological and can give rise to *Seasonal Adaptive Disorder* (SAD), another example of failure to adapt. A successful treatment in some cases is to sit in the glare of full spectrum white light in the early morning. This is similar to awakening with the rising sun. Some people develop all kinds of symptoms as a result of night work because they are unable to adapt to this abnormal life style. It is the versatility of the brain that governs our adaptive mechanisms, and as already discussed, a major cause of failure is poor diet. There are, of course, possibly some cases with genetically determined reasons. The Incas, as part of their preventive medicine approach to life, lay down in the early morning to look briefly at the sun. This was the dose of full spectrum white light that they required for stimulating their adaptive responses.

Heart attacks and strokes are statistically more common in the early morning, related to Circadian rhythm and loss of oxidative efficiency. It is known that rats will develop atherosclerotic lesions with electrical stimulation of the hypothalamus, strongly suggesting that the state of the brain is as important as the state of the arterial system in organic diseases thought to be purely physical. This concept makes it impossible to accept the accuracy of our present disease model and once again illustrates that the brain and body are just two different parts of the same machine.

Love and Hate

The ancient Greeks used three different classifications for love. They called them eros, philos, and agape. The first was applied to sexual love, and the basic mechanics of the sexual act are governed by the limbic system. Cognitive awareness means that a person who is emotionally loved (eros) must be loved in a philos sense to make the relationship a completely satisfying one. True love is a mixture of eros and philos. The top grade, agape, is a pure act of giving. This would mean that the Christian ideal of "love thy neighbor as thyself" is a cognitively directed function which gives rise to actions of charity and selflessness. At the other end of the scale, the opposite of eros is hatred. Some people damage themselves by reacting to the emotion of hatred. I remember a woman who repeatedly attacked her husband with verbal venom like an emotional storm. She developed a typical "stress" related disease that ultimately killed her. As we use more cognitive, controlling power, the two parts of the brain decide the best action to take in response. It is the bell shaped curve of two extremes. The limbic computer is programmed to govern the emotional part of this kind of complex interaction while the cognitive decides the outcome. If the emotion becomes dominant it is at least verging on a form of temporary insanity. Perhaps Hitler was so emotionally filled with hatred that he could be classified as insane by this definition. Some crimes and perhaps vandalism may be due to compulsion as a function of the limbic system without an advisory from the cognitive. A "hot-blooded" crime, such as a murder during the act of rape, may be an act of the limbic brain rather than the cognitive or conscious brain. The "advice and consent" (self control) from the conscious is overwhelmed by the more primitive limbic brain.

High calorie malnutrition appears to create a situation where the limbic brain dominates the cognitive. Thus, a given crime of this nature might be seen as "temporary insanity." Our society is certainly a very long way from even attempting such an idea, let alone trying to see how our law courts could possibly cope with a diagnostic assessment of what sort of crime is represented. Perhaps one day we will be able to distinguish the limbic from the cognitive crime and be able to deal with each in a different way. At present our society is punitive since crime is considered always to be an act of volition. I have already suggested O.J. as a possible example of an "unhinged" but purely temporary state of mind.

Then there is the case of Tucker, the first woman to be executed in the U.S. She killed two people with an ice pick. It was bloody and vicious and there was no doubt at all that she was the culprit. One of the most interesting statements that she made when being interviewed on a national T.V. program was that she experienced several orgasms while she was committing the crime, an obvious reflex reaction of the limbic system.

She became a "born-again Christian" while she was incarcerated on death row. She was reported to be a charming and harmless person who was sincere and would be extremely unlikely to commit any more crimes. She was a drug addict and a delinquent at the time of the crime, suggesting that the limbic brain was responsible. Perhaps her hate for her victims went out of control and the primitive brain was responsible, commensurate with the definition of temporary insanity in the law courts of Ohio. It may be the most intelligent person who is at greatest risk from alcohol, drugs, and addictive tendencies, because a good brain requires the best kind of fuel, just the same as an automobile engine requires the kind of gasoline for which it is designed.

A Nutritional Approach to a Revised Model for Medicine

I published the case of a young African-American man who committed a much less severe crime. As a security guard, he went into a store, showed his gun to the clerk and received a mere twenty dollars from the register. He strolled out of the store and the clerk called the police who immediately arrested him and he confessed. The public defender recognized that this was unusual because he had no previous criminal record and came from a loving family. He therefore questioned his "sanity," as defined in Ohio at the time of the crime and wanted to use that in his defense if it could be proved. We found gross abnormality in the biochemical mechanisms of his nervous system related to his appalling diet. This was corrected with dietary direction and supplementary vitamins and, one year later, he was tested again and the biochemical abnormalities had disappeared. A county judge accepted the evidence at a preliminary hearing and indicated that the public defender could use the "temporary insanity" defense. It was thrown out on appeal to the Ohio High Court by the prosecutor and the young man went to prison. Although his crime cannot be forgiven, the punishment may well have caused him to emerge as a hardened criminal.

The subject of "Road Rage" was published in *Time Magazine* on January 12, 1998. The lead statement was that "aggressive driving is America's sickness *du jour.* But is there a cure for thinking everyone else on the road is an idiot?" It was stated that incidents of "road rage" were up fifty-one percent in the first half of the decade and that some occurrences are grisly enough to make the headlines. Diet was not mentioned because it has not been well introduced to collective consciousness. If a driver is "cut off" by another vehicle, his anger might easily overflow in ungoverned rage if the primitive brain dominates the brain dialogue.

Organic Disease

Although changes are taking place toward diagnosis in terms of the underlying biochemistry and genetic influences, for many years it has generally been considered that each disease has a different cause and that a cure must be found for each one. The concept was derived historically from pursuit of "the enemy," a foreign agent that attacks the body, beginning with the discovery of infecting micro-organisms. If the "attacking agent" is regarded as a "stressor" the ability to recognize its nature is a function of the computer. The ability of the brain/body combination to organize defensive action is the key.

For example, two persons go through an ugly divorce. One of them comes through unscathed and as mentally/physically fit as ever. The other becomes sick with an illness. Was the divorce the cause of the disease? Is stress a cause of anything? Figure 4 shows the relationships in terms of Boolean Algebra, a method of analyzing different influences by means of overlapping circles.

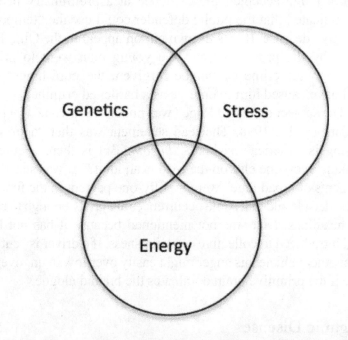

FIGURE 4 *The Three Circles of Health*

Circle One, Genetics

Our parents give us our inherited characteristics through a combination of cellular genes. Our mothers give us the mitochondrial genes that provide the energy that enables the cells to function. Each of us has an almost certain probability of some kind of weakness within this genetic profile. This is the point where a breakdown may occur, perhaps later in life when aging and stress have caused more wear and tear. We know that diabetes can occur after a stress event such as something as trivial as a cold or "flu," or even after reading a telegram that provides bad news. We know, for example that the disease known as *ankylosing spondylitis* is associated with a particular arrangement of genes in the genetic characteristics of an individual. It does not guarantee that such an individual will get the disease. This represents a risk factor and if that person does not obey the rules of diet and life-style, he is more likely to develop the disease.

Circle Two, Stress

This represents the accidental and ever-changing events of living in the world, most of which is beyond our control. We have some choices of course, for we may take a more or less stressful job, for example, or we can decide not to go through a divorce but the choice does not necessarily remove the stress. A person who finds himself in a job that he does not like may not be able to change to another one because of training and experience, or he may find that taking a new job is even more stressful. A person who elects not to go through a divorce may be more stressed by remaining married.

Circle Three, Nutrition

The third circle is the only one over which we have control by providing the fuel that leads to greatest cellular efficiency, metabolic processes that enable energy to be produced in sufficient amount to meet the changing demands. This explains why one person can go through a period of great stress, while another one breaks down and develops a disease. A breakdown in a car is more likely to occur if the engine is stressed by serving it with incorrect fuel.

A middle-aged woman had a life threatening chronic disease known as Wegener's Granuloma. The traditional method of treatment was to administer chemotherapy because it behaves rather like a cancer. She had been treated with chemotherapy and when I first saw her, she was extremely sick, as much from treatment as from the disease. After some months of nutritional supplementation, some given intravenously, she gradually improved. Her health kept breaking down, however, because she had one basic weakness -the craving of sweets. Each relapse would start with one of the symptoms recognized as those associated with her original disease diagnosis. When asked, but never spontaneously mentioned, and even though she was well aware of the association, it inevitably followed from some social functions where she had succumbed to the temptations of sweets. An added problem for her was that there was considerable family stress, a factor that always increases any addictive tendency. Dietary excesses of this nature can overwhelm the metabolic processing of glucose that, for this woman, may have already been marginal for genetically determined as well as dietary reasons. The family stress was an additional factor as depicted in the three circles of health.

Prostaglandins

This is an important part of the adaptive mechanism and has to be outlined to complete the picture.

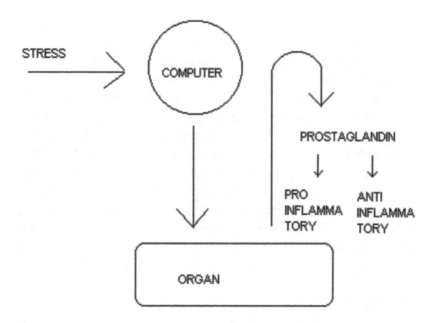

FIGURE 5: *Diagram to show how the signal for inflammation from the computer causes release of inflammatory messengers*

Figure 5 represents an automated reaction that enables us to adapt and survive in a hostile environment. *Prostaglandins* are synthesized in the body from polyunsaturated fatty acids required in our diet. They are similar to the chemical substances that are used by insects to communicate by transfer from one antenna to another in a chemical language. The brain "talks" to the body cells and the body cells "talk" to each other and back to the brain. There are many different molecules produced and they are really modifiers of the action that is required by each of our cells in its contribution to total function. Prostaglandins can therefore be considered as the letters and words of a complex language. The body can be compared with an orchestra where the organ cells are banks of instruments. They are all programmed and know what they have to do. Like an orchestra, they have to be coordinated to "play the symphony of health." Prostaglandins, like many other molecules produced in the body, are messengers and are thus part of the language of communication. They are destroyed quickly after their message has been delivered.

Prostagandins are divided into two large groups known as pro- and anti- inflammatory, although they have many other actions. The two groups obey the principles of yin and yang. One type causes inflammation, while the other one damps it down. We all know that inflammation causes pain. It is easy, therefore, to understand that an anti-inflammatory substance would be logical. Inflammation is a normal and required adaptive mechanism that causes the white blood cells and the nutrients to go to the site of injury. Any injury is followed by inflammation, causing pain, redness and swelling. It is the mechanism that starts the healing process by causing increased blood supply and it is the pro-inflammatory prostaglandins (as well as many other messengers) that can initiate it. It is therefore a defensive process that must be carefully controlled. It has evolved over millions of years. Inflammation that gets out of control is a cause of disease. The proper dietary use of the essential fatty acids used to make prostaglandins is by no means simple since it involves knowledge of very complex biochemistry. It is the skillful use of combinations of these fatty acids that has become an extremely important approach to a whole host of diseases that are not understandable without this knowledge.

The model outlined here makes sense. It provides a rational approach to the difference between health and disease. On many occasions I have given this kind of explanation to patients who have often suffered from disease for many years. They often indicate that it is the first time that anyone has offered a rational explanation for their long term suffering. This becomes more emphatic to them when symptoms gradually disappear over time. It is always important to explain that the leading symptom that is the most important one for them and the major reason for the consultation may be the last one to disappear. The other ones, often taken for granted and accepted as part of their constitution, are the ones that clear up first.

CHAPTER 6

HOW THE MODEL APPLIES TO THERAPY

The model proposed here is reductionist, implying that we are little more than chemical machines. It has been said that we are more than that, involving the concept of spirit and soul, both of which are unknown entities. We still know little about the cognitive brain and how it is able to do complex thought processes. We do not have any idea what "free will" is or how it is engineered. The lower, primitive brain is a complex computer that governs our ability to adapt to environment. We have compared this computer to a radio where the volume of sound it produces can be controlled. Emotions are accompanied by physical changes in the body. What good nutrition does is to regulate the intensity of the response, equivalent to reducing volume in a radio.

Nutrition: Prevention and Therapy

Our present approach to a large part of our nutrition is hedonistic, meaning that it gives a jolt of pleasure. Our food should be aimed at eating and drinking the fuel that makes the cellular engines run efficiently. We have evidently lost the "body wisdom" that enables wild animals to discern the food that they should seek that is not harmful. Mother Nature produces poisonous substances as well as those that provide us with food. Deadly Nightshade, a common weed, is a good example. Nutrition is the most important factor in maintaining health. Some people are becoming more sophisticated on this subject and have done their own research in pursuit of their own health and that of their families. Physicians of the 21st century will be expected to be able to educate their patients in the right choices of food and the food supplements that have become an important factor in both maintaining and retrieving health.

Why supplements? The food industry and modern farming practices make sure that we have lots of calorie producing food without the essential vitamins and minerals that enable the calories to be used efficiently.

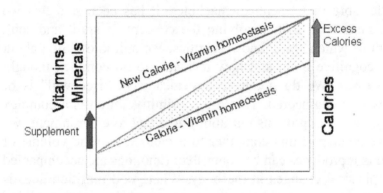

FIGURE 6: *How empty calories (the dotted triangle) upset the calorie/vitamin ratio*

The most obvious foods that are detrimental are the sweet simple carbohydrates. For many people who are sugar sensitive it must be discontinued totally in order to ascertain whether sugar is the culprit. Non-caloric nutritional supplements do not work unless the offending foods are withdrawn.

As one example amongst many, I saw a child who had been treated for severe temper tantrums, attention deficit, and tics. He had a history of birth trauma that compromised his limbic computer through oxygen deficit. His maturation was delayed and he was experiencing abnormal reactions to input stimulus.

A Nutritional Approach to a Revised Model for Medicine

By withdrawing all the junk foods and providing him with supplemental nutrients, his maturation began to catch up with his chronological age. The tics and temper tantrums disappeared and he became much more cooperative commensurate with age. One of the withdrawn foods was cow's milk and although this might surprise many people, the father told me later that if even a tiny amount of milk was given to him, he would "go completely out of control."

Milk is almost an untouchable item of "health food" whose nutritional properties have been artificially fanned, mainly because of its calcium content. It is dollar driven and the taste factor is of great commercial concern. I sometimes find children who cry when they are told that they have to give up milk. It is possibly stretching it to say that they are addicted, but they certainly crave it. So ingrained is the notion of nutritional benefit from milk in the minds of most mothers, that they are shocked when they are directed to discontinue giving it to the child in question. They invariably ask, "Where is the calcium going to come from"? on the mistaken assumption that milk is the only source of this element. Milk is a natural food that is provided by the mother of any mammal for her infant after birth. It is a temporary food until the infant has teeth. The human is the only species that takes milk of another mammal as a diet staple. Its withdrawal from the diet of many children is beneficial and may result in a dramatic change in personality and behavior as soon as five days after withdrawal. Bovine growth hormone and antibiotics are given to cows to increase milk production and prevent mastitis. Both of these drugs are ingested and may play a part in the unwanted reactions caused by milk.

A common cause of ill health today is coffee, already emphasized in a previous chapter. Caffeine is a stimulant, particularly to the limbic brain, so that any incoming stimuli may trigger a reaction that would not otherwise occur. Many different kinds of reflexes, such as runs of sneezing, spasmodic coughing attacks, palpitations of the heart, or irritable bowel action may be initiated. An individual who has become addicted to caffeine may be maladapted to daily life stresses. The problem is that the constitution of each of us is unique and may or may not make us more susceptible to the action of any drug including sugar and coffee. The symptoms described are usually attributed to those of a specific disease entity such as allergy. For instance, a patient of my acquaintance had suffered from a spasmodic cough for two years. She had been investigated repeatedly for pulmonary disease because it is automatically assumed that coughing of this nature is caused by lung disease. With dietary changes and non-caloric supplements, the cough disappeared. The mechanism was an exaggerated reflex due to increased sensitivity of the limbic brain. One of the clues to this is that coughing often occurred during sleep without awakening the individual.

Another source of confusion is that, in most people, there is often no immediate symptomatic reaction in response to drinking coffee, although some may notice heart palpitations or a sense of nervousness. When there is no immediate effect there is no awareness that they are gradually inducing reactivity that makes them susceptible to other forms of stimulus. The drug is simply setting them up. Sneezing and coughing are protective reflexes to provide an explosive mechanism designed to get rid of a foreign substance, a normal part of the genetically determined hygiene of the body. Sensory input to the computer triggers the normal reflex motor phenomena that make all the necessary components go into action because of sensitivity in the reflex control mechanism. Thus there may be spontaneous episodes of sneezing or coughing for no apparent reason. The feeling of overcoming fatigue by drinking coffee is deceptive. It is taken by many people in the morning to give them the "energy" to face the day. It stimulates action and actually consumes cellular energy that may well be already in short supply. The sense of action from it gives the impression that it is "needed" but it is merely stimulating brain action in the release of neurotransmission: hence the expenditure of energy and the consequent possibility of feeling "let down." When coffee is discontinued, it may give rise to headaches, often very severe, and these are typical withdrawal symptoms that occur after withdrawal of virtually any addictive drug. It is true that coffee contains antioxidants but their benefit is frequently overcome by the ill effects of caffeine.

Acupuncture

This treatment has been around for at least 5,000 years and it may be that it came into being a great deal sooner than that. It is unlikely that it would have been a spurious form of treatment to last all this time. The ancient Chinese, as we have already discussed, discovered that there were channels of communication throughout the body that they called meridians. They believed that acupuncture restored the "state of balance" represented in the concept of yin and yang, possibly by unblocking a stream of energy flowing through the body/brain. There is good evidence that this is correct in terms of our increasing understanding of the brain/body association. When the autonomic nervous system is balanced, homeostasis is restored because we are at rest. The sympathetic and parasympathetic branches of the system are activated as a means of adapting to a given stimulus. The brain /body combination is really in a state of *homeodynamic equilibrium*. Acupuncture seems to be a way of stimulating the brain computer. It also appears to connect the input stimulus through the interconnecting meridians to other organs, carrying information that has to be data processed. We know, for example, that there is a marked increase in endorphins from the brain during acupuncture, a discovery that was published from research done in England. Endorphins are substances that are produced naturally in our brains and have a variety of different effects. One of the major ones is to damp down the way in which our brains perceive the input signal that gives rise to pain. We know, also, that the technique of acupuncture can be used to produce anesthesia that is so efficient that a surgeon can open the chest or remove an appendix when used on a patient.

Perhaps acupuncture stimulates the weak side of an imbalance to restore homeodynamics, as do nutrients. Calcium and magnesium, vital participants in cellular machinery, must be in a balance like sodium and potassium, zinc and copper and many other nutritional elements. Every adaptive emotional and physical reaction is a temporary state of imbalance, or yin versus yang. If a depressed person were to be treated successfully with acupuncture, it would be a demonstration of restoration of balance between the various brain chemicals and a return to the normal intermediate resting state of homeostasis when everything is in balance. The computer calls for an adaptive reaction of the whole organism to meet a given stimulus. Depression is the opposite of euphoria. Sweating is the opposite of shivering, both of which are adaptive reactions to changes in temperature.

Some years ago, I was confronted with the case of a child whose symmetry of adaptive responses had been physically changed by the nature of her diet. The phenomenon for which her mother brought her was ostensibly "emotional disease." She had violent temper tantrums. During them, one half of her body would become pink on one side and white on the other. It was as though a line had been drawn down the middle of her body mindful of Harlequin. In addition, one pupil in her eye would dilate and the other would not. She was studied in some detail and it was found that she had asymmetric adaptive reactions dictated by the brain computer. More sweat could be obtained from one arm than from the other. The electroencephalogram (brainwave test) was different on the two sides of the brain. The blood pressure was different in one arm as compared with the other. Dietary correction and a few nutritional supplements were initiated and she was tested again one year later. All the former asymmetry of reactivity had disappeared and she was no longer having her temper tantrums.

The brain governs each half of the body separately and in this girl the asymmetry was greatly exaggerated and unbalanced. Some asymmetry is quite normal. All of us have one foot slightly bigger than the other or one eye a bit more open than the other. Breast size asymmetry is very common. There is a rare congenital condition in which a child is born with one half of the body bigger than the other. Even one half of the head is bigger and two limbs are longer and heavier on one side than the other. It probably illustrates that the electrical potential delivered from the central brain computer guides the growth and development of the body as it passes through the complexities of embryonic development. Thus, the brain is in charge from the very beginning of our development. If the electric messages are stronger on one side than the other it is possible to postulate that it is the original cause of the asymmetry, the organs growing in response to the strength of the stimulus. It has long been known that the autonomic nervous system controls the two halves of the body asymmetrically although the reason for this is unknown.

Homeopathy

Homeopathy was founded in the 1790s by the German physician Samuel Hahnemann. He developed the law of similars by testing various substances on himself. This was based on the principle that "likes are cured by likes." Drugs or medicines that cause disease symptoms in healthy individuals can also be used to cure illnesses that produce the same symptoms in sick individuals, according to this principle. A patient studied in this manner is given a medication that has been found to cause the symptom, but it is given in a vanishingly small dose. For example, if a person has been found to suffer from arsenic poisoning, a minute dose of arsenic is administered. This obviously disagrees with the medical model of today.

The principle depends upon stimulating the body's defense whether it is reacting to a live microorganism or a foreign chemical. There is some evidence that the water that carries the remedy has a "memory" of its own and can become "electrically imprinted" with the "memory" of the substance dissolved in it. With excessive dilution as is used in homeopathy, the memory remains. Thus, a substance that is dissolved in water and then diluted to the point where the original substance could not be detected, carries information to the brain because the water carries the memory of the substance that was dissolved in it and then diluted to non-existence. This stimulates the body to recognize that "an enemy is within" and that it must mobilize its defensive resources, much in the same way that immunization works.

A developing test procedure is performed by assessing the "electrical balance" of a person by measuring it at the acupuncture sites on the hands. A computer then determines whether the balance is "low" or "high." An appropriate homeopathic remedy is calculated by the computer and the requisite dilute mixture is given in the form of drops that are taken by mouth. Nutrients can be examined also in the circuitry attached to the patient and used to "restore balance." As with nutritional therapy, a homeopathic remedy may cause the patient to have a temporary increase in symptoms, followed by gradual improvement. I have seen this happen in a patient who was totally unresponsive to all the nutrients and other remedies attempted previously.

A research group in Hungary has been studying the art of homeopathy and its scientists believe that they have found proof that it is scientifically sound. Their proof, however, is delivered in mathematical terms, so that the non-mathematical mind cannot understand the language. An American trained physician in Taiwan has been studying homeopathy for years and has carried out experiments that have shown close diagnostic agreement with traditional laboratory methods. She uses a machine that is hooked up to acupuncture points on the patient's hands and feet and the electrical information that is generated from the patient's energy sources is passed into a computer. The energy "balance" is assessed by the computer and a course of action dictated without a single blood test or any other invasive phenomenon.

This is hard to understand in the light of our present medical model. Our culture, in general, does every possible thing to make sure that health preservation is neutralized by our diet, our beverages, our life style and excessive business stress. Homeopathy and acupuncture are natural cousins and it is logical to see them in a state of cooperation. Both can be seen as a form of input stimulation.

Biofeedback

This is a valuable technique in treating conditions that are conventionally considered to be psychological or psychosomatic. By the use of specialized electrical devices, the patient is taught to control the autonomic nervous system voluntarily. The cognitive, upper brain is exercised to overdrive otherwise automatic body functions. Although some automatic mechanisms such as breathing can be voluntarily controlled, biofeedback simply extends that principle by increasing the influence of the cognitive over the automatic nature of the brain computer.

As an example, ulcerative colitis tends to affect intelligent people who are experiencing mental stress. In the view of many physicians, the disease is considered to be purely physical without considering the role of the brain whose input is frequently denied because of many abnormal laboratory tests that indicate organic disease. It is impossible to understand the action of mental stress unless the brain computer is taken into consideration. The damage to the bowel is inflicted by complex actions originating from it. Biofeedback is very helpful in this disease and supports the role of brain in its etiology. Nutritional therapy, provided at the same time by making the brain computer more logical in its adaptive responses, does much the same thing and is an essential part of treatment.

Derrick Lonsdale M.D.

As an example, an intelligent woman in her thirties had ulcerative colitis. Her job was extremely stressful and her personality was very deceptive. On the surface, she appeared to be very calm and relaxed, although in reality she was a compulsive perfectionist. Nutritional treatment met with only partial success but, with biofeedback, she began to make real progress. Malabsorption from the bowel, due to the inflammation, had induced Vitamin K deficiency that caused bleeding. When this was added to her nutrient regimen the bleeding ceased and there was a dramatic improvement in all aspects of her health. Obviously, there was a combination of brain computer drive and tissue nutrient deficiency. Vitamin K is now known to be involved with many different aspects of body chemistry and has even been found to be part of bone metabolism, so it is a useful supplement in the prevention and treatment of osteoporosis, together with Vitamin D.

It is an example of the fact that health is made up of many different components that must fit together like a jig-saw puzzle. It is interesting to note that it was a combination of dietary correction, use of appropriate supplements, and biofeedback that was necessary. One method alone was insufficient.

The most modern biofeedback techniques involve the use of the *electroencephalogram* (EEG) and Siegfried Othmer, Ph.D. wrote an article entitled "EEG Biofeedback Training" in the *Journal of Mind Technology* and I quote from this article. He wrote that Kamiya, as long ago as the sixties, found that EEG activity could be altered deliberately by means of feedback of EEG information to the subject. A researcher by the name of Barry Sterman at the UCLA School of Medicine was doing sleep studies with cats in the late sixties and found that a certain rhythmic activity was present in both the sleeping and waking state. He was successful in training that activity as well, with the consequence that he was able to manipulate the sleep state in the animals, He became aware that brainwave training could change behavior and it launched a lengthy period of research.

It was found that seizure incidence, intensity, and duration could be reduced in humans with EEG training. The technique has, however, remained in the view of orthodoxy, highly speculative and unproven so that few physicians are using it.

The article stated that many conditions can be treated successfully by this method, including traumatic brain injury, some stroke patients, fetal alcohol syndrome, attention deficit disorder, depression, and even dementia. The author mentions the treatment of a number of conditions that are traditionally considered to be emotional in the Freudian context. Many of the conditions referred to by Dr. Othmer respond to nutrient therapy. In combination with biofeedback, they do a better job than either one performed separately.

A patient of my acquaintance had suffered daily headaches for fifty years. He could not remember a single day that he was free from this scourge. Nutrient therapy failed to help him and he was referred for biofeedback. He became free from headache in one month. What was uncovered by the biofeedback training was the fact that this gentleman's problem was locked into a state of internal tension of which he was entirely unaware. He was also taught the art of meditation and, since then, he has become so good at this discipline that he can do it in any place that he chooses and at any time that he pleases.

Massotherapy

This is a relatively new form of treatment, using massage. Massotherapists have a specialized curriculum of training that is widely different from that of physiotherapists. They know where the "trigger points" in the muscles are and their massage involves the whole body, not just the part that is the localized source of the patient's muscle pain and stiffness. It is an extremely soothing technique when administered by an expert and can be accompanied by very softly played music, creating a situation that is almost hypnotic. There is often immediate relief of pain from the common condition of *fibromyalgia*, though it usually comes back slowly over a few days and the treatment then needs to be repeated. As the therapist continues to repeat these treatments, there may be permanent or long lasting relief. The "physical" is the same as the "mental" as the two inevitably work together. Fibromyalgia is related to tension and psychological stress in some people and it may well be that the effect of massage is not too different from acupuncture by sending sensory stimuli into the brain computer and causing it to become more balanced in its adaptive strategy.

The effect of the computer on the muscular system is illustrated by considering the condition of scoliosis, where the vertebral column gradually becomes more curved, concave to either the left or right. The spinal column is maintained in its rigid state partly by the muscles that are attached to it on either side. These muscles are kept "in tone" which means that the muscle fibers are receiving a continuous bombardment of signals from the computer in the brain. Tone means that the muscles are maintained in a permanent state of tension that enables them to act as supportive columns on each side of the spine. This tone can easily be appreciated by placing a hand on the back, particularly in the lower part or lumbar regions. They feel like steel bars more than muscles. The fact that we can move the spinal column as we bend the body in our daily lives is due to the fact that the tone can be relaxed or voluntarily overdriven. That means, of course, that the brain must engineer relaxation of muscles on the left side of the vertebral column when the body bends to the right. The "tonic signals" continuously received by these muscles are directed evenly on either side of the spine under normal circumstances. In the formation of scoliosis, the signals are delivered more strongly to one side than the other, thus slowly causing the column to become bent. As already discussed, the computer can deliver signals that are asymmetric in the two halves of the body. An exaggeration of this asymmetry is disastrous. One of the complications of a genetically determined disease known as *Familial Dysautonomia* is scoliosis, the reason being that the mechanism of this disease is caused by a disturbance in the brain computer.

The conventional treatment for scoliosis is a back brace or surgery. Another treatment that has been tried is to fit electrodes into the nerve supply of the muscles on the convex side. This stems from the fact that these muscles are weaker than those on the concave side and continuous electrical input to these muscles gradually restores the balance that results in straightening of the vertebral column. On completion of this, attention must be paid to the internal mechanism of the original cause of asymmetry. This can be achieved by restoring normal metabolic processes involved in cellular energy synthesis through nutritional therapy.

Drug Therapy

The pharmaceutical industry rules modern medicine. Almost daily, a new discovery about the intricate details of disease mechanism is announced in the media. In nearly every case, the researcher who has made the discovery is interviewed and the statement that is usually made is repetitive. "This discovery may lead to the formulation of a new drug that will have an effect on this mechanism." It is a promise that has fallen flat countless times. Drugs, particularly synthetic chemicals, are inevitably foreign to the body and are instantly recognized as such. The first thing that the body attempts is to break down the chemical components of the drug and get rid of them. That is why the drug has to be taken at intervals during the day in order to maintain its effect.

Pharmaceutical drugs act only during the time that they remain intact in the body before the natural mechanisms break it down. Another very real problem is that many of its effects during this active period are unpredictable and even unknown in many cases. Sometimes the metabolic products are toxic or have pharmacological effects that are unknown, giving rise to the well-known phenomenon of "side effects." It is always instructive to read about virtually any drug in the *Physicians' Desk Reference,* the book that is now almost as large and heavy as the traditional family bible. The chemical properties are first described. Its pharmacological action comes next and is quite frequently described as "action unknown." A short paragraph follows, in which the doses and various details of prescribing are outlined and then there are often several pages of potential side effects. If the average patient took the trouble to read about the prescription it would not be filled in many cases.

The February 8 issue of *Newsweek* in 1999 provided some statistics on drug use in America. The article was entitled "Screening for Genes" and began with a story of a nine-year-old boy who was treated for leukemia. The child belonged to a small group of the population who carry a gene that leaves them unable to metabolize a whole family of drugs. One of these is a thiopurine that is prescribed for childhood leukemia. Because, as the article continued, his doctors did not check him for the gene, the drug "wiped out his bone marrow" because he was a "mismatch between his genes and the medicine meant to save his life." Under the heading "Prescription of Disaster" the article noted that more than 100.000 people die in the U.S. every year because they carry "misspelled" genes that make medication either ineffective or deadly. "Now" it continued, "doctors can test for the genes before prescribing," and a list of drugs is given and the effect of them in a person with this genetic inability.

If the drug is to be used and an expensive test is required before it is to be safely administered, should it be used at all? Conventional medicine says that drugs are a necessity, and the only way to approach the problem. Since healing is a function of the body, we should be working hard to learn more about providing nutrient assistance to help the natural process safely and effectively. Ritalin is used in treatment of a whole array of conditions in children. An article in *Time* magazine that was issued on November 30, 1988 was introduced by a picture of

A Nutritional Approach to a Revised Model for Medicine

a child on the cover and the heading, "The latest on Ritalin: Scientists later said that it works. But how do you know if it's right for your kids?" The article itself begins with "What exactly does a normal child look like?" Its title is "The Age of Ritalin."

A family therapist, who has written several books on raising children, was quoted as saying "but why does it work, and what are the consequences of overprescribing? The reality is we don't know." The use of this drug is so widespread that the country actually ran out of it a few years ago. That means, of course, that there are literally millions of children that are being treated this way. I have talked to teachers who tell me that they had perhaps one of these affected children in the class thirty years ago and now they have between ten and twenty who have varying degrees of attention deficit, hyperactivity, and learning disability. I cannot see how we can fail to draw the conclusion that there is something wrong with our environment in causing such a disaster. It is impossible to believe that Mother Nature made this many genetic mistakes, but that is a common interpretation. Another major disaster is portrayed in this article under the heading of "Next Up: Prozac." It continues "When you're ten years old, you shouldn't have much to be depressed about or so an adult might think. But just as more and more children are taking Ritalin to calm their hyperactivity storms, a growing number of kids are turning to Prozac and other antidepressants to treat their blues."

Time magazine reported that there were about 3.4 million Americans under eighteen who are said to be depressed, in a state of biochemical imbalance. The suicide rate is on the increase. There has to be something very wrong with brain chemistry to lead to suicide. I talked to a patient that had experienced depression. I asked him whether he had ever been suicidal. He said that he had, but he was quite unable to determine why he had ever thought of it at all. "It was as though another person inside me was dictating the idea."

A study of a popular drug for depression was compared with the action of St. John's Wort, also a popular herbal remedy. A third "arm" of the study was the use of a placebo, always used in drug studies. The drug and the herb came out about even. It may be a surprise to know that the placebo came out on top! The study cost six million dollars. It is absurd to sneer at the placebo effect. If we knew how it worked and could "turn it on" at will, we would not need any "treatment" of any sort. It is an example of the "power of the mind" over the purely physical aspects of the body.

Autistic Spectrum Disorder

It is now considered by many physicians that the epidemic of autism represents the upper end of a spectrum of mental disorder in children. Many of the most severely affected children may have an unusually good cognitive mental ability that cannot be expressed. For example, I have encountered parents who say that their autistic child can perform on the home computer better than they can. They are usually aware that their child is unusually intelligent and perceptive behind the façade of disintegrated behavior. It may be that this intelligence puts them at risk. A good brain requires a colossal amount of energy to run it and that means that oxygen is consumed at a fast rate. If that oxidation mechanism is allowed to become inefficient, the brain activity will become distorted and that means that behavior will be different from what is expected. It may be that the brightest and the best are in the greatest danger. Just the same as the highly tuned racing car engine needs superior fuel, so do these children require superior nutrition. Our failure to recognize that and the failure of our society to appreciate the fundamental dangers of our food industry, together with the imposition of a highly polluted world, represent our collective failure.

At the lower end of the spectrum (ASD), affected children are given a diagnostic label like attention deficit, hyperactivity, or Tourette Syndrome. An analogy would be variations on a symphonic theme. They are not different disease entities. Because of an unknown genetic risk (the genetics circle) these children appear to be born on a "metabolic cliff." An environmental stress factor (the stress circle) "knocks them off the cliff." This may explain why some children succumb to vaccinations, antibiotic abuse, and other multiple stress factors while others do not. Observation of children within this spectrum strongly suggests that they are immature for their chronologic age. Much of their activity, including their devastating temper tantrums, is limbic (the brain computer) in character because the hard wiring of the brain has been retarded. Some children in the higher functioning lower end of the spectrum can focus when they (mostly boys) become fascinated or interested in something, as in taking blood pressure during the physical examination. The blood pressure is a sensitive way of judging the state of imbalance in the computer, and the child often will pick up the bulb on the blood pressure machine and start pumping it. He is inquisitive and wants to see what happens when he does this. As he performs this action he becomes quieter and focused.

By removal of the high calorie "junk foods" and providing some vitamin supplements, the overall intelligence of the child usually begins to emerge. He begins to sleep at night as children used to sleep. The temper tantrums gradually disappear as maturation proceeds although the time that it will take for normal brain balance to be restored is unpredictable. I have seen extreme hyperactivity disappear in five days, just with the removal of milk from the diet. But I have also seen it take as long as two years, suggesting that the brain chemistry is much more severe and harder to reach.

Full blown autism lies at the high end of this spectrum and is usually associated with permanent damage to brain function that cannot be reached by any means. We can expect the best results if the autistic spectrum is recognized early enough in infancy but there are signs that are being ignored by many pediatricians. The very first suspicion must arise with jaundice in the newborn. This is treated with ultraviolet light and is explained as "physiological." The second phenomenon that should raise our suspicions is the behavior called "colic" where the infant draws up his knees and screams, sometimes day and night and sometimes just between the evening hours of six and ten p.m. These two effects are almost certainly induced by sickness in the mother during pregnancy, the commonest being nausea and vomiting that goes throughout the pregnancy. It has been published that this known technically as hyperemesis gravidarum is associated with deficiencies of B group vitamins. The third phenomenon that needs to be spotted is repeated ear infections. It starts with the infant crying and sometimes "pulling at his ear." At this early time the ear drum is inflamed and red in color. If the inflammation is eased with ear drops containing a little hydrocortisone and an antibiotic, the inflammation will disappear. If not, then bacterial infection ensues. Most histories of children in this spectrum include the appearance of repeated ear infections that lead to antibiotic abuse and are a very important sign of worse things to come. It has now been published that newborn jaundice and the behavior of the infant known as "colic" are both indications of "oxidative stress" (loss of efficiency in the use of oxygen in synthesizing cellular energy) and are important symptoms to recognize. It is so easy to put an infant like this on a well rounded vitamin therapy for it may well be an act of prevention.

Stress

A middle-aged woman gave the following story. About ten years previously, she had experienced a pain that began in the right shoulder and radiated across the front of her chest and abdomen into the left hip. She had visited a physician who had found gallstones. It would be accepted by any physician that they were the cause of the pain and her gall bladder was removed. The only problem was that, after the surgery, the pain was exactly the same as before.

If the gall-stones were the original cause of the pain, and shoulder pain can certainly be related, perhaps the sensory message became a source of input to the brain computer where it was stored as a "file" in the "hard drive." Any form of physical or mental stress thereafter was an input to the "hard drive" and the "file" came up on the "monitor" to reiterate the pain that she had experienced ten years ago and for which the original cause had been removed. By correcting the diet and providing some nutritional supplements the pain had disappeared within a month. This is perhaps why a person that has been abused in childhood retains a powerful unconscious memory that might be compared with a file in the hard drive of a computer.

Faith Healing

This requires a belief system that transcends self. The case of a young native in Africa who had offended the local witch doctor can be used as an example. The witch doctor shook a bone in front of the face of his unfortunate young victim and told him that he would die. He started to become gradually more sick and was taken to the westernized clinic where everything that was attempted was to no avail. He continued to lose weight and was in the process of gradually dying. Finally, in desperation, the western doctor called upon the witch doctor and asked him to consider taking the curse off his victim. When he agreed to do it, he simply shook the same bone in front of the man and told him that he had been forgiven, whereupon the patient immediately began to recover. The power invested in the witch doctor is in the minds of the people that he serves. The modern American physician does not possess this power. He is considered to wield scientific tools that may or may not work. There is no power invested in him as a healer, perhaps because we are either more sophisticated or more cynical in our ability to believe in anything that we cannot ourselves perceive. A person who has intense and irrevocable faith takes it for granted. It is indeed a rarity in this day and age, but the witch doctor is still a powerful "deity" in his own right and is viewed by his "patients/victims" as having special powers. It is surely the nuts and bolts of religious belief and it matters little whether the substance is scientifically beyond proof. There is no surprise when it works. Perhaps faith causes the brain to focus the healing resources of the body into the tissue compartment where the disease process is at work, resulting in a concentration of that healing power. A cancer cell is seen for what it is; a maverick cell that has broken the laws of cooperative cellular function and it is duly destroyed as it would be under the most healthy life-style. Generating that power demands something that is generally perceived as miraculous. Something, or someone, outside and above ourselves is seen as possessing that power. If we destroy the phenomenon of that blind faith, the power is removed. It is worth noting that a miracle is something observed that has no explanation. If its mechanism is discovered, it ceases to be a miracle.

It is this mechanism that is responsible for the need to perform the "gold standard" test procedure of the double blind study for testing the efficacy of drugs. It has been recognized for years that a drug may work only because of the faith that the patient has in being subject to its effect. A placebo is a "dummy" that looks just like the real thing but has nothing in it that can possibly affect the physiology of the tested subject. Unconsciously, the person is influenced by the fact that he truly believes that the pill that he is taking is the real thing. A successful drug is considered when there is a statistically significant difference between the benefits experienced from the real drug as compared with the fake. If the results from each group are the same, the drug is deemed to be a failure. In some cases, the side effects of the drug may create a situation that is worse than those who received placebo. If we could accurately harness the placebo effect in every sick person, we would not need potentially dangerous drugs. It may be that nutritional therapy assists the placebo effect, focusing the faith factor by providing the required energy.

Sometimes a physician, even in today's world, can help in such a manner. I remember Brenda who, at the age of seventeen years, had cancer that spread through her entire abdomen. She was treated in the conventional way with chemotherapy and, a month later, she had to be readmitted with complications that appeared to be hopeless. One day, Brenda's parents were sitting in her hospital room crying and broadcasting their sense of hopelessness. Brenda was lying with her face turned away toward the wall, the very model of "giving up." It was suggested to the parents they should try to show a feeling of optimism, whether they felt it or not. Brenda was quietly told that she could not be helped if she gave up. On the next day Brenda asked when she could go home. She was told that she could leave at once because there was no evidence that her bowel was obstructed by the cancer and she could continue with her therapy.

During the ensuing year Brenda became the very spirit of optimism. She delighted her fellow students in high school and would spend the evenings making cookies that she took to school for her friends. Every time that she returned for follow up visits she always brought a wooly toy animal that she had made herself. I still have them, years later. Brenda died about a year later and, even today, her case might be considered unusual by the standards of expected response. Although, in that case, I certainly was not given the power of the witch doctor, perhaps I acted as a catalyst that enabled Brenda to focus on things outside herself. Perhaps this held back the process, at least for a time that would not otherwise have been available to this family. I mention the family, because the people that surround a sick person are just as important as the medicines that are provided. Let a physician who believes that he has affected a cure ponder the real issues. He may well be congratulating himself instead of the patient!

In the present medical model, physicians are taught to be "aggressive" to destroy the disease or keep it under control. . Also, if physicians really listen to what their patients have to say, they often spill the vital clues. It might be compared with a jig-saw puzzle where the pieces have to be found and fitted into the picture.

CHAPTER 7

OPPORTUNIST ORGANISMS

A person with an infection such as "the flu" goes into a room where there are twenty people. He coughs and sneezes over all of them and perhaps only five or six get "the flu." We all know, of course, that this is because the defenses of the five or six are insufficiently strong to cope with the viral attack. The others are immune because their immune systems are strong enough to protect them from this particular organism. This is really true of all potentially pathogenic organisms. Each makes an attack and has to create a "beach-head" within the tissues of the host. The host must sense the presence of the potential predator and become alert to the necessity of its own defense. Staphylococci are common infecting organisms. If they gain a hold on someone by coming into contact with a cut on the skin, the first thing that happens is a local alert warning that results in a rush of white cells toward the foe, in much the same way as a locally stationed militia might act if a foreign army came ashore.

When the staphylococci begin a battle within the "beach-head," many of the defending white cells die and become pus, forming a boil or pustule. They have, as it were, sacrificed themselves on behalf of the whole organism. If the attack is quenched at this point, the pustule will gradually dry up, or it may discharge the purulent material and heal. If, on the other hand, the "beach-head" is not contained, the staphylococci may invade the lymphatic system, causing *lymphangitis,* or pass directly into the blood to start a *septicemia.* At this stage, it is

A Nutritional Approach to a Revised Model for Medicine

"all-out war" and the entire system of the victim is mobilized. The body temperature is raised and the bone marrow is "ordered" to make millions of white cells, the "defensive soldiers."

Before the days of antibiotics, a state of affairs like this was often lethal and still is if antibiotic resistance is encountered.

Perhaps the story of a schoolboy illustrates this attack/defense phenomenon in the pre-antibiotic era. He was changing for soccer in a room with a wooden floor and received a large splinter in his foot. The injury became septic and began to invade his body through the lymphatic system. The family doctor immediately recognized the danger and ordered his mother to tear up some old blankets into strips and boil them. As soon as the strips of blankets had cooled enough to avoid scalding, they were wrapped around his leg from thigh to foot. Some delirium accompanied the high fever that followed. Within a day or so a "crisis" occurred when the infection had been contained. The treatment was simply designed to make it more difficult for the staphylococci to "win the war." By encouraging a rise in local tissue temperature and the ensuing rise in body temperature, the natural defense mechanisms prevailed. All the microorganisms that are capable of attacking us are really opportunists. Perhaps those potentially infecting ones that surround us are merely "testing agents." If we do not obey the rules and weaken ourselves in our ability to adapt within the natural world, they may be our only predators in keeping with the Darwinian concept of "survival of the fittest."

When pathogenic microorganisms were discovered we started to look for ways and means to kill them without killing the infected patient. Even our approach to prevention through immunization has some drawbacks. For example, pertussis (whooping cough) vaccine has caused its own health problems in some. The triple vaccine MMR (measles, mumps and rubella) has been called into question as a possible cause of a number of children to become autistic. The vaccine for hepatitis B has been made compulsory in many states and there is evidence that it may have caused some health problems. The introduction of hepatitis B on day one after birth is a tragic mistake. An infant relies on the antibodies derived from his mother for what is known as "passive" immunity. He is not capable of mounting his own "active" immunity until he is three months of age.

The search for adequate means of killing these predatory microorganisms led to the discovery of penicillin and our entry into the antibiotic era. As we ignore the rules set by Mother Nature, we seek artificial means to defend ourselves from the consequences of infection without considering why the attacking organisms win the war. Civilization has provided us with ever increasing convenience that has led us to believe that we can ignore the fitness of our own body defenses.

A rise in body temperature is a defensive mechanism which is "ordered" by the brain computer. This is because bacteria have their most lethal effect at 37° C, the normal body temperature. We are once again reminded of yin and yang since we do not want the body temperature to be either too low or too high and it is at the intermediate level when we are healthy. Artificial reduction of elevated body temperature in infection is counterproductive and many people will remember that there was a condition that occurred in children and adolescents called Reye's Syndrome, an acutely lethal disease which appeared to come in winter epidemics. It took us a long time to become aware that we were actually producing the disease by administration of aspirin to reduce fever in an otherwise non-lethal, self-limiting condition that would not have been dangerous to the patient if it had been left alone. Although thousands of children received aspirin for their relatively trivial infections, it is true that only a few of them contracted Reye's Syndrome. This is due to the biologic variability of all human beings.

Under ideal circumstances, the "thermostat" in the brain will reset the body temperature to go up in order to "cook" the invader. It is true that if the body temperature becomes too high, it can cause adverse effects but this may occur because

A Nutritional Approach to a Revised Model for Medicine

the brain computer is in a state of biochemical dysfunction and does not do its thermostatic control properly. Perhaps, because of poor diet, or a long period of "stress," or from a combination of factors, a person might be energy depleted when the infection occurs and the natural defenses too easily overwhelmed. The computer organizes body defenses and, if it is electrochemically damaged, it will not perform the necessary adaptive program. An excessive increase in body temperature from a disordered control mechanism is the opposite of no such response, the yin and yang.

To cite an example of this in my experience, I admitted a middle-aged man to hospital with pneumonia. I was a resident in my teaching hospital in England. In an English hospital, at least in those days, the ward was a large room that contained twenty or thirty beds for men only and the same for women. He was well known as a long-term patient because he had tuberculosis and the pneumonia was an acute overlay to his existing chronic disease. In the morning, my chief came into the hospital ward where this man could easily be observed from just within the ward door. He quietly pointed out the dying patient. He had noted that the patient was picking with his fingers at the bedclothes. Occasionally he would reach out and pick at thin air. He went on to explain that this meant that the patient's brain was so intoxicated by disease that it was reacting entirely automatically while he was otherwise unconscious, a phenomenon well known to experienced physicians.

To me, the information was so completely instructive that I have remembered the case in vivid terms, even though it occurred some 60 years ago. The laboratory data were all normal. There was no elevation of body temperature, no increase in the white blood cell count, nothing to indicate imminently lethal disease. At autopsy, this man was found to have *staphylococcal* abscesses throughout his entire body. He was literally riddled with millions of these pathogenic organisms. He never would have survived, even today.

Derrick Lonsdale M.D.

The point is that this unfortunate man had been slowly but surely deprived of any ability to mount defensive measures against an attack of this nature. We know that tuberculosis is itself caused by an opportunist organism and chronic malnutrition had led to total decay of his immune response. The modern counterpart of this would be the overlay of tuberculosis in a patient with AIDS. It is extremely important to see the role played by the brain in this example of a death from overwhelming infection.

The only time that I have seen this phenomenon again was when I was in family practice. One evening, I was asked to perform a house call. The patient was a middle-aged man who was in the "all fours" position on a double bed. The only light in the room was shed by a bare blue bulb hanging from the ceiling. As I entered the room, his clouded and seemingly unresponsive eyes looked directly at me and he reached forward to "pick at thin air," the same phenomenon described above in the other patient.

He died in hospital and was found to have meningitis that had been caused by a *pneumococcus,* an organism that is frequently responsible for pneumonia. He had been suffering from a cough that his family had failed to recognize as serious. He had an unrecognized pneumonia and the organism that caused it had spread to cause lethal meningitis. This case, like the previous one, was of a person whose immune system had been wrecked, probably by years of poor diet.

This emphasizes again that potentially pathogenic microorganisms are "opportunistic." An infection, as all of us have at times, is really a test of our defensive mechanisms. They only become dangerous when these natural defenses are weakened. The brain computer organizes the immune mechanisms and it is erroneous to talk about the immune system as though it were an autonomous mechanism that occurs specifically in the body without its organizing action.

We keep hearing about "new diseases" caused by an ever-increasing list of dangerous microorganisms, many of which are viruses. The organisms are not new; they have always been here. It is unfortunate that we fail to think in "attack versus defense" terms when we consider these organisms, the only predators that we have since we are at the top of the food-chain. It is not too hard to see why we are becoming weakened. Our lifestyle is contrary to that which was set for us before civilization began. I am not advocating a return to our caveman days, I am only saying that we should remember the principles of our natural origins as members of the animal kingdom.

Healthy people do not succumb often, if at all, to infections because they have adequate energy developing mechanisms in all of their body cells. The health of the limbic system is crucial since it has to organize the defense. If we really went about the business of health in an appropriate manner, we would actually abolish the use of the physician as we know him today. Perhaps this process has already begun as the general public is finding out that good nutrition is a major factor. Sometimes a patient may know more about this than a physician and is quite shocked when the physician indicates that "taking those vitamins is a waste of time and money." I do not wish to leave the impression that taking supplemental vitamins "takes us off the hook" of self responsibility. The primary thrust must be in determining an appropriate diet and complete removal of the high calorie "junk" that is so prevalent in the world of today.

It may well be that we are actually making things worse for ourselves by the abuse of antibiotics. It would seem to be logical to assume that there is some kind of ecological relationship between bacteria and viruses, since there is a pattern to all of natural existence. There seems to be an increasing virulence to viral diseases and it is conceivable that we are actually strengthening their power to attack us by upsetting this ecology through the abuse of antibiotics. It is, of course, impossible to tell whether this is really so, or whether it is our own defensive weakness that is at the root. I know that my clinical experience has been that many of the patients with chronic fatigue syndrome started out with an acute episode of "flu" that was treated with an antibiotic. Recently, I became aware of an individual who had his common cold treated with one of these increasingly dangerous drugs. He nearly died as a result of its side effects.

Another important point is that patients often expect an antibiotic to be prescribed and the physician is, in a sense, "blackmailed" into using one of these drugs. If the patient gets worse, the physician's defense in a lawsuit is that he prescribed an antibiotic. Defensive medicine is all too common and is a major cause of increasing cost.

Some time ago I became aware that a convocation of experts was being convened to discuss formulation of a vaccine aimed at ear infections. This means, of course, that there is a general realization that "ear infections" are in pandemic form in our children. This is, in my opinion, the worst possible way to address the situation. It is unnecessary and, if such a vaccine is ever produced, it might be as potentially dangerous to some children as the ones that we already have. By improving the nutrition of the child and adding a few simple nutrient supplements, ear infections do not occur. The ear mechanism in a child is made of tissue that is extremely active from a metabolic standpoint. It requires a disproportionate amount of oxygen and nutrients to carry out its twenty-four-hour schedule of hearing. It is metabolic decline that provides opportunity to the bacteria. Thus, the infection is secondary to inflammation caused by a release of inflammation-causing eicosanoids, described in an earlier chapter. It is important to recognize that inflammation is organized and directed as a defensive mechanism that must be initiated by the limbic brain. If this mechanism is excitable because of metabolic inefficiency, the result is a signal that results in an unnecessary defensive reaction that is itself abnormal. Bacterial infection often follows. I once asked an audience of parents, all of whom had at least one child with autism, "How many of you experienced repeated ear infection in your child before his autism was recognized?" About two thirds of the audience raised their hands, indicating that this was a common phenomenon in the early history of a child who is already on the way to developing a condition that is now known as Autistic Spectrum Disorder (ASD). This is called a spectrum because it is now thought by many researchers that there are a number of disorders that have previously been considered as distinct entities. These include the high functioning child with Attention Deficit, Attention Deficit Hyperactivity Disorder, Tourette Syndrome and varying degrees of dysfunction, such as auditory processing, at the bottom end of the spectrum. Autism, with low functioning, is the severest at the top end. Thus they are all due to biochemical changes in various parts of the brain and with varying degree of severity. I have already mentioned that it has recently been published in a medical journal that jaundice of the newborn, treated by exposure to UV light or sunlight, and "colic" are the first signs of oxidative stress in an infant. And like recurrent ear infections, should now be regarded with great respect in terms of a preventive approach. Both of these are common parts of the history in a child who appears at the age of three to five years with the obvious signs of ASD. The sooner a knowledgeable pediatrician sees such a child and recognizes these important signs, the better are the chances of preventing the disaster that is so prevalent in the children of today.

Children are experiencing these drastic changes in health, largely because of atrocious nutrition involving an excess of sugar in particular. Because most physicians fail to take in the attack/defense issue, the only thought given to it is how to "kill the enemy," the bacteria that are considered to be the primary cause. As the antibiotics become stronger and more aggressive, the child's metabolism is more and more at risk.

The history is so often the same in the ultimate diagnosis of ASD that it is almost predictable from case to case. The first clinical problem is that the infant, commonly a boy, often has what is usually referred to as "colic." He is irritable and cries constantly, although in some cases this is only between the hours of six and ten p.m. In many infants it is twenty-four hours a day and I have seen a situation where a mother has not been able to obtain a full night's sleep in as long as two years! Naturally, this is very disruptive to the family as a whole, the father often interpreting the situation as inadequate mothering skills.

One day, about the age of seven or eight months, the infant perhaps pulls his ear when in a state of irritability. The mother takes him to a pediatrician, particularly if there is an associated fever. The pediatrician, seeing an inflamed eardrum, makes a diagnosis of an ear infection and the child receives an antibiotic. Now begins a series of such incidents that occur repetitively over the next few years, driving the family into a state of total frustration. At about the age of four years, the child is referred to a surgeon who sticks little tubes through the eardrums. The parents are often told that these are drainage tubes, but their real benefit is obtained by allowing air, and hence oxygen, to enter the ear cavity. Sometimes, even this does not always stop the infections and the child goes from pediatrician to allergist to surgeon for removal of adenoids and/or tonsils. Finally, when the child goes to his first kindergarten assignment, the teacher calls the mother and says that she cannot handle the child. He is unable to sit still or his attention span is too short or he is actually disruptive to the class. The ultimate classification stuck on the child is Attention Deficit Disease (ADD) or one of its variants.

The infancy "colic" is a symptom arising from an irritable brain. This may arise as a result of the mother's diet during pregnancy, or because of his cow's milk ingestion. Infantile jaundice and "colic" are the first signs of oxidative stress and both of these are extremely common in forecasting autistic spectrum disorder. Pulling his ear and crying may be an indication of pain or part of his expression of irritability. If there is fever, it is worth remembering that it is produced by the brain computer and may well be part of the expression of irritability. The inflamed eardrum seen by the pediatrician is due to inflammation produced by the internal mechanisms already described previously. Infection may follow because the inflamed area provides a good culture medium for bacteria, but it is not the original cause. The problem can often be solved in the early stage by the use of ear drops containing a little cortisol and antibiotic. The mother can easily keep some of the ear drops at hand and can administer them if she suspects that an ear inflammation is arising. Since this often happens in the night and the mother is awakened by her child crying, it can be a simple expedient that prevents ultimate infection. The child usually settles down and goes to sleep fairly soon.

The main thrust of treatment; however, is to make sure that dietary causes are removed. Supplementary vitamin/mineral preparations make the nutritional needs complete and the recurrent episodes soon cease.

What has this got to do with the later onset of ADD? This is a very important question since the pandemic of this condition in the United States is widespread. There is some evidence that it is the repetitive use of antibiotics that is at least partly responsible. The damage may be from the destruction of friendly (symbiotic) bacteria in the bowel, with subsequent appearance of a bacteria/yeast imbalance. Worse yet may be the mechanism of damaged mitochondria as described in a previous chapter.

Yeast

Many people are now aware of an organism that has made significant differences to their health. The best known yeast that affects humans is *candida albicans*, but there are a number of yeasts that are less common that can infect us. They are all essentially opportunist and *candida albicans* is particularly notable since it is sometimes referred to as the Jekyll and Hyde Organism. A number of books have been written on the subject of *candida* infections and it is fairly well known to many people, particularly women because they suffer from vaginal infections from this organism quite commonly. The *Candidiasis* Syndrome that is common today is totally rejected by mainstream medicine unless the immune system is severely compromised as, for example, in AIDS. This is the reason that it has been characterized as opportunistic. It will only take a hold in the human body if there is a depleted defense system. What most physicians believe, however, is that the immune system must be so damaged that the patient's life is in danger. They have not accepted the fact that this kind of infection can be associated with common disorders that abound in the American population today.

The syndrome is an extremely frustrating one because of the unusual nature of the *candida* organism which is normally symbiotic, meaning that it performs duties for the host in whom it lives. Its function is recycling organic material, exactly the same kind of function that it has in nature as a whole. If the yeast detects an ecological breakdown in its environment within the bowel of the host, it changes its form to become *mycelial*, meaning that it begins to spread in the typical method of any mold. The commonest cause of the breakdown is the use of powerful antibiotics that wipe out many of the symbiotic bacteria upon which so much of our digestive processes depend. This results in a bacteria/yeast imbalance. The *candida*, detecting the imbalance, becomes a predator. At the ends of the *mycelia* capable of growing through the bowel wall, spores develop and will emerge as new *candida* organisms. The spores can travel in the bloodstream to other parts of the body where they colonize.

To say that the bowel of a person is "moldy" is not far from the truth and it can be seen that the "headquarters" of the offending organism is within the bowel. Depending upon the seriousness of the person's defense systems, the *candida* might be confined only to the bowel, or it might grow through the bowel wall and get into the body's system, when it is known as "*systemic candidiasis.*" There is a rare condition known as *muco-cutaneous candidiasis* that occurs in infants. Because of some inborn error in the normal defenses against this organism, the yeast grows on the skin and on the mucous membranes. It usually starts with "thrush" as an infant and continues unabated as the child grows. It was not until the drug called ketoconazole was synthesized that any form of treatment was available. This medication kills systemic yeast and is valuable when the body system has been invaded.

In the case of a girl, a still unidentified substance that appears to exist in serum from normal people was absent in hers. Something had gone wrong with the normal ability of the body to synthesize this undefined, but vital substance that is produced as a specific defense against the predictable invasion by yeast. The highest concentration of it is known to exist in the conjunctival fluid that bathes the eyes of cows. This is ecologically sound since mold would be expected to occur in cow fodder and affect its eyes without this protection. Human blood serum is a good culture medium for both bacteria and molds and it is not surprising that we are normally equipped with a defense of this nature. Perhaps the easiest way to encourage the growth of yeast in the bowel is by the ingestion of sugar since this is used in the alcohol fermentation process.

One of the byproducts of wine making is tartaric acid and this has to be removed or nobody would drink the wine. When yeast invades the human bowel and ferments dietary sugar, tartaric acid is formed and is absorbed and excreted in urine. Thus this can be detected in a specimen of urine from a patient suspected of yeast infection. In the current epidemic of autism in children this test is frequently positive and subsequent treatment to kill off the offending bowel yeast sometimes results in major clinical improvement. Some children with ADD have been found to have this substance in their urine. This supports the contention that antibiotics, commonly given as indicated above, may have a great deal to do with the widespread appearance of this affliction.

The characteristic symptoms of yeast vaginitis are itching and a typical discharge. It is usually treated with a locally applied remedy, without considering the primary reason. The symptoms clear up by this means, but quickly return on completion of treatment because the underlying cause has not been addressed. It is generally conceded that this infection arrives by direct spread from the bowel, but it may be blood borne in some cases. Many afflicted patients have Pre Menstrual Syndrome (PMS), or Chronic Fatigue Syndrome (CFS), many will have Tempero Mandibular Joint Syndrome. (TMJ), and or Mitral Valve Prolapse (MVP) Syndrome, all of which are associated with dysfunction of the autonomic system. The statistics for all of these conditions are very troubling because they affect so much of the American population.

Treatment

It must be readily apparent that to "kill the enemy" without improving the host defense mechanisms is a waste of time and effort. Much of the cause of *candidiasis* is iatrogenic (doctor produced) by the often unnecessary use of increasingly powerful antibiotics and perhaps even other drugs. Sugar ingestion is frequently a major associated cause. Thus, lifestyle and appropriate nutrition are the main considerations. Supplementary non-caloric nutrients are important, but do not work well without addressing the main sources of poor diet. Nystatin is an antibiotic that is specific for dealing with yeast in the bowel. It is not absorbed and has no effect on the normal bowel bacteria. Various medications based on the original ketoconazole are prescription items that deal with systemic yeast infection

E-B Virus

E-B stands for Epstein-Barr, the cause of the so-called "kissing disease" or mononucleosis. It is called the "kissing disease" because it is relatively common in adolescents and is considered to be infectious. After a test for E-B was found, we were led to

A Nutritional Approach to a Revised Model for Medicine

believe that we had a diagnostic test for mononucleosis. After a little while, it was found that this test could be positive even in healthy people and its diagnostic message was muted. Now, we are aware that the concentration of the antibodies to the virus increases rapidly when a person has the symptoms referred to as mononucleosis, sometimes called "mono."

We have to conclude that the E-B virus can be found, as it has now been estimated, in ninety to ninety-five percent of the population. Obviously this huge population is not sick from the disease. What is now believed is that the virus is acquired at some time in life of nearly all of us and awaits its opportunity. It appears to be capable of detecting when the immune defenses have weakened sufficiently to give it a chance of winning the war, an example of the balance that exists between predator and prey. It is hardly surprising, therefore, that young people with an attack of mononucleosis are ignorant of the basic reason why they have succumbed. It is because at that age, within our modern culture, "junk" food and beverages are all too common. They are at school or college and their days are crammed with a rush of activity called "burning the candle at both ends." This requires sufficient cellular energy that must be derived from diet.

Providing nutritional counseling to such an affected individual often fails. We have come to accept the fact that the virus is the cause of the disease and that we have no responsibility towards ourselves in being affected by an affliction of this nature, or any other infection for that matter. It is always a constellation of circumstances that come together, the infecting organism as the potential predator, a period of stress that causes excessive energy utilization, and the quality of nutrition. It is a balance between attack and defense. The only valuable method of treating mononucleosis is by supporting the altered chemistry of the victim with improved nutrition. There is no satisfactory method of killing the virus by artificial means. The usual antibiotics are ineffective on viruses. Non-caloric nutrients given by intravenous administration results in the patient getting back to school or work within a week or so instead of what may be as long as three to six months. The excessive fatigue, sore throats, and swelling of lymph glands are all related to how the brain computer is failing to organize the defensive mechanisms of the body in an appropriate and logical manner.

Streptococcus

I have already suggested that all microorganisms are opportunistic and I am reminded of a particular family. There were four children, all very bright and active in their daily lives. Their mother had accepted the disease model described here and was particularly careful about diet and nutrition. In spite of this, one of her children would occasionally succumb to a proven strep throat. It invariably occurred on the day after the child had been to a birthday party. It seemed as though the streptococcus was "waiting in the wings" and we know, of course, that an organism like this can reside in the throat without causing illness. Such a person is known as a "strep carrier." It is tolerated but not rejected as a foe or even a potential foe. Something has to happen to activate the organism to attack. Apparently, the streptococcus was activated by the kind of "food" that is traditional at birthday parties. Why was it that these particular children succumbed when others at the party did not? Therein lies the question that has fooled us for too many years. Humans are uniquely different and we each have weaknesses and strengths that differ in an endless variety of ways. The child would have to be a carrier of the streptococcus and that is, in itself, a weakness. These bacteria should not be tolerated at all as residents of the throat. Something else would have to happen in order to activate them and make them cause an infection. The birthday party was stressful enough to make this activation possible.

I asked the mother what she thought that she ought to do about the "junk" that is an automatic accompaniment of birthday parties. They represent the social life of children and she pointed out that she could not call the host mother and request that her child be served appropriate natural foods against the traditional fare. She had decided that the risk had to be taken anyway, for the obvious cultural reasons. It is not an indictment on the mother or how she was raising her family. It is an indictment on our culture that does not accept the principles of good nutrition. It depends upon a number of accessory factors that include the constitutional fitness of the child from a genetically determined standpoint and the rate at which a child like this is developing both mentally and physically.

We do not know exactly why a streptococcus is tolerated in some individuals. We have to assume that the carrier state would not be tolerated if the nutrition of the child was ideal. Less than ideal may be enough to fail in generating the extra energy for the growth, development, and individual activity of a rapidly growing child. The "junk" food becomes the "last straw to break the camel's back." Thus, the birthday party is only part of the cause and cannot be solely to blame. Putting poor fuel into an engine only creates poor engine performance. A growing child needs pristine, balanced nutrition to meet the accelerated cellular energy demands that are automatically required. If this is done and the child receives a few vitamin supplements, he no longer suffers from this kind of recurrent infection. He has grown up and outgrown the accelerated demand of physical and mental development. Of great importance in this biologic equation is the fact that each of these children are intelligent and extremely active in numerous social and school activities. It is the most intelligent children that are most at risk. Couple an active brain with rapid growth and fuel consumption can be expected to be proportional.

One of these children, a boy then in his adolescent years, was brought back to see me. The symptoms were mostly in terms of his behavior, but on the physical examination I found that his blood pressure had increased. He had some of the stigmata of poor nutrition and I told him flatly that if he wished to go out for something like football or other athletic endeavor, he might very well be turned down on the necessary sports physical that would be required. I made it clear that his inattention to appropriate dietary rules was the cause of all his symptoms and he left my office with sufficient fear that he actually did listen to what his mother had been trying to tell him about his diet. I saw his mother some months later and asked if the boy had changed at all and she was happy to report that he had. Sometimes the advice of a physician is better accepted if a would-be athlete is told that his athletic performance would improve. It is no accident that good athletes are better academic students, assuming of course that they apply themselves.

Another factor may be what is usually called idiosyncrasy. This means that the effect of a given substance on a child might be devastating for that particular child, as a unique individual. We know that certain food dyes, particularly the yellow and red ones, will cause fundamental and critical behavioral changes in some children. Conventional wisdom says that this is impossible but each person is uniquely different from everyone else, living, dead, or yet to be borne.

"New" Viruses

We keep hearing about "new" viruses that are responsible for some devastating and frequently lethal diseases, such as Ebola. They are probably not new and may also be opportunistic. Even the HIV virus which causes AIDS may exist in a person for years before the disease appears. It may even be possible that a person could acquire the virus and never become sick from it? Possibly, this would be logical if the defenses are vigorous enough and maintained. Perhaps because of malnutrition, profligate lifestyle, emotional trauma or other forms of stress, the adaptive machinery is overwhelmed. It is true, of course, that a truly new organism might emerge and that there is no immune memory in anyone for this organism. It is thought that Ebola, for example, is a new organism to humans because it has emerged from the rapidly disappearing rain forest and jungle. Another example is the Myxoma Virus that was introduced into rabbits in Australia and other countries. The total lack of immune response to this genuinely new organism caused an epidemic that wiped out most of the rabbit population. When an immune response began to appear in the animals, the population recovered.

Herpes

There are two different organisms that are responsible for this kind of affliction. One of them causes "cold sores," painful blisters around the mouth. The other causes similar lesions in the genital area. Both are opportunistic. A gentleman of my acquaintance would develop a "cold sore" every time he played tennis on a sunny day. Since ultraviolet rays are stressful to the body, that appeared to be the factor that triggered the infection. It had to mean, of course, that the infectious agent was always there and became active only when the host was stressed in this particular manner. The same thing applies to its appearance in many people when they are infected with a cold virus. Genital herpes erupts repeatedly after sexual intercourse. The amino acid, lysine, taken in sufficient quantity as a supplement, will either protect an individual from recurrent outbreaks or can be used to treat one when it occurs, another example of assisting the normal protective mechanisms of the host.

Sun tanning is a protective mechanism that prevents the action of ultra violet rays in producing sunburn. It is also sunlight that enables us to make Vitamin D. For this reason good health is necessary to develop a tan rather than the other way round. Before the antibiotic age, tuberculosis was treated in sanatoria by exposing the patients to sunlight in the open air. Perhaps it was the rest and the better food that were the most important features of the treatment since we have reason to believe that it was not medication but better living conditions, better nutrition and better hygiene that almost abolished tuberculosis. We are now finding its reemergence in people that have depressed immunity, as in AIDS victims.

All our medical resources are aimed at protection from the environmental hazards that surround us. As drugs become progressively more potent in order to kill the resistant bacteria, they become more dangerous to us. It is a vicious cycle similar to the problems that have arisen in modern agriculture where more and more chemicals are used to kill the pests. Their development of resistance causes the need to find yet another chemical. Antibiotic resistance is now a major hurdle, particularly in the treatment of hospital acquired infections.

CHAPTER 8

CASE ILLUSTRATIONS

There was a very good reason for my personal change in concept. I was educated in a British medical school where the training was based upon the teachings of Sir William Osler. When the modern era of medicine in America was ushered in, chiefly by the dictates of Rockefeller following the "Flexner Report," the principles were based on the German concept that the laboratory was the ultimate guide to a successful outcome of treatment. Osler, who was then at Johns Hopkins, was the leading clinician of his day and had concluded that observation of the patient was the most important aspect of diagnosis. He disagreed with the laboratory-based methodology that became the platform on which our present day medicine is based. He immigrated to England where much of the training in medical schools was derived from Osler's teaching. I learned about people and their every-day complaints and problems, and much less about the detailed science that is the basis for function in the body. That came later, but the most important aspect of clinical medicine is the whole person who walks into a physician's office.

In short, we were trained to see the patient as a whole living being. The general appearance and observation of small differences became second nature to us. I have absolutely no doubt that this approach should be more encouraged in American medical schools. I have observed that many medical students graduating from them are much too dependent upon laboratory findings which are often accepted at face value. The general appearance of the patient is not as much taken in as it should be. Furthermore, the training appears to be didactic enough that it is difficult to escape from the rules set by the lectures of their professors.

Like most physicians, I have evolved on the basis of hard-won experience. Medical school provides basic training for the job and you then start to learn. Before the mandatory residency posts, you have to make a career choice. The two major divisions are surgery and medicine and then whether or not to take a specialty. I liked it all, but I knew that I didn't have the right personality for surgery and I aimed myself at being a family physician.

Until the arrival of the British National Health Service, family practice had been almost exclusively private and then that changed dramatically. A family physician became a slave to the whims of the patient and I became acutely aware of how amazingly selfish and manipulative people can be. But it was marvelous experience and I certainly learned a great deal about patients and the diverse way in which they present their problems.

My first practice engagement was in a small town in Suffolk. It was very much a country practice and we spent most of our days making house calls to country cottages within about a ten-mile radius of the town. As in most country places, a stranger had to "become accepted" and everyone was suspicious of a new doctor, often being under the impression that it represented a substitute for the "real thing."

Country people do not mince their words. They are forthright and direct. They are also extremely stoical in the face of suffering.

One summer evening, I took a house call in the country. Addresses of cottages were always a mystery since they were tucked away down small country lanes and numbering was virtually still in the "space age" to come. When I found it, I was confronted with a young woman who was in shock from a ruptured ectopic pregnancy and she was bleeding internally.

A Nutritional Approach to a Revised Model for Medicine

Having given her an injection of morphine for the shock, I raced back to the village to direct the ambulance to the house and we took her to the cottage hospital where her abdomen was opened by a surgeon while I administered the anesthetic.

I can still remember the case as though it happened yesterday. The surgeon had set up an open container in which he had placed a gauze filter and the container was connected to an arm vein in the patient. He scooped out masses of blood in the abdominal cavity and dumped it into the container, thus providing the patient with her own blood, filtered through the gauze. Not only did she recover very quickly, she never had the slightest sign of any kind of reaction such as fever and there was never any indication of infection.

This case made me acutely aware of the extraordinary resilience of the human body if you can do things for it that do not actively cause harm. This woman avoided the risk of receiving someone else's blood and was nurtured in her own home locality where she was known to so many people. Today, she would have a preventive antibiotic that would be another risk factor, as we have already discussed. It was truly amazing to see how well these country people did with the kind of crude care that we were able to offer.

Another example was a middle-aged man who had no less than three or four heart attacks. With each one, I took care of him in his own home, paying house calls on a regular basis. In those days, we had no idea that such a thing as a heart attack could be related to diet, but it was quite an acceptable thing to treat it with rest and relaxation, something that the modern hospital does not properly address. Today, this man would have had one or more bypass surgeries and would have been in an intensive care unit, surrounded by all the frightening events happening to other patients and with all the noise that seems to be an inevitable factor in hospitals.

This must cause us to pause and wonder how much our high powered and expensive technology has improved the lot of seriously ill people. Intensive care units had not been invented, even in large hospitals. It is tacitly accepted that we invariably do better today than we did then, but I have seen the most appalling disasters that could be logically ascribed to the treatment of the patient rather than the disease. Of course, there are many exceptions and, in a surgical emergency, certainly give me the technology of today, as long as I am not turned into a vegetative state because of it.

It is not necessary to discard our gains but it is vitally necessary to use them wisely. I was made acutely aware of how this can be manipulated to the detriment of all on the basis of power structure and politics based upon the belief of invincibility often possessed by modern surgeons. I knew a gentleman who was paralyzed from the waist down, due to poliomyelitis. He was, of course, wheel chair bound. His wife had to help him with virtually every physical challenge, although he had an excellent brain and was very perceptive and intelligent. One day, he had chest pain that was interpreted as a heart attack. His family doctor put him in a local hospital and requested the help of a cardiologist to treat him medically. Both of them considered surgery to be indefensible.

The president of the company, for which my friend had worked until his retirement, stepped into the situation. He was a local "big wheel" who knew a well known cardiac surgeon personally. The company president insisted that my friend be moved to the hospital where this surgeon operated for bypass surgery. No doubt he felt that his influence was a great asset. Anyway, the surgery took place and my friend was then cared for in the Intensive Care Unit. After many weeks of anguish for his wife and family, his life just ebbed away, and he died without ever leaving the ICU. To anyone with judgment, the outcome was predictable. It should have been obvious that this man was an exceedingly poor risk for surgery, to be sacrificed to macho influence, and unwise posturing of this nature.

The point that I am trying to make should be obvious to all. The "high tech" mentality has affected the structure of medicine to the point where surgeons in the large medical institutions often conclude that they are almost infallible. Granted, their technical skill for sewing tubes together is incredible, but that is only a means to an end. They do not carry out the process of healing. They merely line up the cut tissues and the body performs the healing. They sometimes forget that this is an energy consuming process where the necessary energy may be quite inadequate to meet the super-stress of surgery in a patient who is already sick. If the treatment is worse than the disease at which it is aimed, then it is better to leave the disease alone. It is more logical to help the healing process by providing the right environment for the patient and giving the nutrients that are required to create the increased amount of energy needed.

Let me take another example of surgical stress at its worst. For a number of years, I worked with a physician who headed a large clinical laboratory. He told me the following story.

Every now and again, a surgical patient would have a rapid and dramatic fall in blood cholesterol after the surgery was completed and would eventually die. This can be explained only by using the stress model that I have outlined in a previous chapter. When a person is under stress as in surgery, the "alarm bells" in the body ring. The computer then sends a message out that will govern all the defense reactions that are needed. It is automatic and is a normal reaction. The adrenal gland is responsible for synthesizing a whole series of hormones known as the "stress hormones" which are secreted into the blood stream as part of the "fight-or-flight" reflex that we discussed earlier. These hormones are constructed from cholesterol that is, in turn, synthesized in the liver. In a massive surgical assault on an already sick patient, energy metabolism is depleted and is insufficient to replace the cholesterol used in the process of synthesizing the hormones needed to meet the stress and the patient dies in shock.

Obviously, the blood cholesterol declines as it is used up and not replaced. It is, however, obvious that it is not the low blood cholesterol that kills the patient. It is a failure of the whole system to mobilize the energy required to meet the stress. The blood cholesterol is merely an effect of this and can be used as an indicator of the impending disaster. It would be logical, therefore, to nourish the patient properly before surgery is ever performed. In some cases, that might even be sufficient to avoid surgery altogether.

Clinical judgment in such a situation is more important than all the "high tech" in the world. Surgeons sometimes fail to take into account the stress effect of the operation and judge the patient to be sick because of the fact that a body organ that he plans to remove is the cause of the illness. Actually, the diseased organ is the effect of the illness, not the cause. It is originally a biochemical storm in the organ that leaves it damaged and often beyond repair. Surgery then becomes a regretful necessity and that is why surgery is an admission of medical failure.

The present medical model labels each and every disease with a name category where the next step is to try to find the correct drug to combat it. Each disease is considered to be a distinct entity in its own right. The names given them are often purely descriptive and are based on a constellation of symptoms and observations made on patients. Research is aimed at finding a specific cure in the form of a medication. This model is the natural sequence that follows the discovery of micro-organisms as already discussed.

Every condition is more or less regarded as an enemy to be defeated. The physician is seen as "being in control" of that process by the supposedly skilful use of medications, the actions of which are often unknown. This general perception is illustrated by the often repeated question; "what vitamin should be prescribed for disease X?" The answer is in finding the underlying biochemical and electrical failure and then applying the appropriate nutrient that will enable the affected tissues to create their own energy to give rise to healing. Thus, different diseases, as they are classified today, may have the same biochemical underlying cause, while different biochemical abnormalities may give rise to the same disease. Two diseases may have to be treated with the same nutrients since they both have a common biochemical cause. A condition like rheumatoid arthritis can have many different nutrient approaches in different people.

The fallacy of our present model arises from the Newtonian concept that we have to identify the millions of different mechanisms that the body possesses naturally to repair itself. We then spend all our research resources in trying to patch the broken part rather than asking the question of why it broke down in the first place. The only possible way to treat energy deficit is through nutrient support. The new model indicates that the symptoms, at least in the initial stages of the disease process, are like "alarm bells" ringing in a complex system. They do not necessarily give you any idea as to what is causing them. To treat these symptoms by blocking them with a drug is superficial and does nothing for their cause. A few examples might illustrate how addressing the biochemical cause is much closer to the mark.

Nutrition is really common sense. We were designed to eat the food that was supplied by Mother Nature. Our ancestor hominids were hunter-gatherers and had to seek their food in the forest. We established agriculture some ten thousand years ago so that we could raise the food at our greater convenience. It has been more or less downhill ever since, so that now we drive a two ton machine to a supermarket to buy food in boxes, again for our convenience.

Hippocrates is still regarded as the "Father of modern medicine." During the 20th century, this has been ignored in practice. He put his patients to rest, gave them adequate and appropriate nourishment, caused the playing of soft and tranquilizing music, and waited for the self-healing process. Unfortunately, we have come to believe that ancient practices have been replaced by scientific miracles. It is considered that

Hippocrates could do little else since he did not have any of the modern techniques and diagnostic equipment that we have today. It is much the same as our attitude has been to traditional Chinese medicine that has been in continuous practice for at least 5,000 years and is unlikely to be fraudulent when seen in its historical context.

One of the patients who taught me to think beyond my medical school lectures was a six-year old boy. His mother brought him in because of a two-year history of recurrent illnesses. Each of the illnesses was similar in nature. First, he would become irritable and his face would become pale. He would complain of a sore throat and develop fever which rose rapidly to about 102 to 104 degrees. Naturally, he would be taken to a physician and, inevitably, would receive an antibiotic on the basis of it being caused by infection. He had been investigated in many places, including prestigious medical institutions, and no physician had ever found a germ, virus or any other microorganism that was responsible.

This is a very common event in pediatrics. It is usually referred to as *fever of unknown origin*, or F.U.O. and is always investigated in terms of seeking the source of the infection. The patient was admitted to a hospital for detailed studies. The mother said something to me that became a most important factor. She asked me to check the level of folic acid and Vitamin B12 in his blood. This seemed to be a most peculiar request to make in the face of the apparent problem and I asked her why. She explained that the child had been in a major hospital where studies had been carried out and that the doctors had found elevated levels of these two vitamins in his blood. She told me that they had criticized her because she was giving the child too many vitamins.

She was unable to understand this because, although she denied giving him any vitamins, they refused to believe her. The two vitamins were found to be in a very high concentration in the child's blood. This was very puzzling because there was no precedent. How could there be any form of connection between recurrent illnesses of this nature and high levels of two B group vitamins? I found evidence that his system was short of Vitamin B1 and found some credible evidence for the association. Vitamin B1 was given to him in fairly large doses and he was sent home.

On his return visit to the clinic he had remained well with no recurrences of his feverish illness. Blood levels of folic acid and Vitamin B 12 were in the normal range. I then asked the mother to stop giving him Vitamin B1. Although she was reluctant, she agreed to do it in the interests of science and to try to obtain proof that her child was at last on the right track. About three weeks later, this child had a night terror and started to sleep walk down the stairs. As he did so, he urinated involuntarily. Then he developed a fever, sore throat, and a huge swollen gland in his neck. The mother brought him back and the blood levels of folic acid and Vitamin B 12 were again elevated. Vitamin B 1 was again administered and within five days he was well again. The folic acid and B12 vitamin blood levels were again normal. He continued to take only Vitamin B1 as a supplement. One year later he began to develop similar episodes and the addition of a multivitamin/mineral complex supplement solved the problem. It exposed an extremely important fact that is constantly being forgotten. Vitamins do not work in the body as single agents. They are not to be used as one might take an aspirin to relieve a headache. They function in a complex team relationship with all the other vitamins and minerals that the body requires to run its machinery properly.

Although this was a most unusual case, I have since learned that it is not a rare incident since I have seen other similar cases. It is necessary to distinguish between a phenomenon of this nature and a true bacterial infection where an antibiotic is required. It is so bizarre in terms of present concepts that it was considered to be an unacceptable explanation by my colleagues. It happened that there was a student who was unusually interested in it and wished to understand it better. He was one of the older students and had run his own contracting business before going into medicine, so he was more mature in contrast to those that had come straight out of college. He did his own research and then presented the case with the associated biochemistry to his fellow students and residents. There was not a single question raised by the audience and it was clear that they rejected it completely. It is sometimes said that there is nothing as successful as success itself, but in this case the success could not be seen by the other students as rational. Even with an explanation as provided, they were unequivocally hostile and unaccepting. I had experience with another case similar to this and published the two case reports in a relatively obscure medical journal. One of the bigger, mainstream medical journals would never have accepted it because vitamin therapy was rejected. I have never received a request for a reprint. Any article in a medical journal is subjected to peer review, and this can sometimes act as a censorship. If the reviewer has the dogmatic view that "vitamin therapy is quackery," he will consciously or unconsciously refute the arguments within the article, irrespective of the beneficial outcome for the patient. I have had a number of papers refused because of this censorship.

The traditional explanation would be that this child had undergone a *spontaneous remission*. This means that there is no explanation for it and it must remain a mystery. None of my staff colleagues asked me about it and it was tacitly assumed that it was simply an unknown event with a false explanation. It is surprising to think that physicians can ignore something as dramatic as this because it conflicts with previous teaching. You would think that they would want to discuss the underlying nature of the phenomenon to see how it could be developed in similar situations. It is hardly surprising that progress in the science of medicine is slow. Of course, we do not wish to publish work that has no worth. That is why peer review was established in the first place, but it is also easy to see that it can be a "two-edged sword."

A Nutritional Approach to a Revised Model for Medicine

For me, it was as much of a turning point as anything could have been. I can still see the face of that boy and his young mother, because they have been etched into my memory. But, from the long haul, it made me wonder whether we were on the wrong track much of the time in our modern medicine. How many other children have suffered the same fate where the illnesses were simply passed off as recurrent attacks by unknown germs?

How does this fit into the model described in a previous chapter? Well, it can only be answered by a hypothetical explanation but so many things have been changed by intuition and it is often true that science catches up later. I concluded that the situation was as follows. I had already discovered that the brain computer becomes much more irritable when there is something as important as a defect in Vitamin B 1 metabolism. The nature of its irritability, however, is either "emotional, physical or both," the decision occurring in the automatic mechanisms of the brain. In this case, there was an "emotional" component expressed by irritability. The fever was initiated by the computer on the basis of being a false alarm. It was "under the impression" that an attack was under way and it was preparing the defense reactions as it would do if a germ or virus had actually been the attacker. The swollen glands were part of this defense also, something that would be expected if a bacterial or viral invasion had actually occurred. There is also another possible explanation. Perhaps it was indeed an attack by an unknown virus which was "waiting in the wings." Such opportunist organisms only attack us when we are in some way weakened. By far and away the commonest cause of that weakening is high calorie malnutrition, particularly in many of our children who are exposed very early to "junk" food.

The point is, however, that it was the computer brain that was initiating each of these episodes, whether there was a real or a spurious attack causing them. The deficiency of effective Vitamin B1 had affected its reactivity, initiating a reflex defensive mechanism. The computer functions according to its processing of sensory input.

This is not an automatic indication of Vitamin B1 deficiency. The same reaction can occur because of a deficiency in any one or more of the total vitamin spectrum that each one of us needs. It is the loss of efficiency in the metabolic processes of the brain that is the true cause. Any one or more of the vitamin and mineral team can cause a similar exaggeration in maladaptive responses of this nature.

On another occasion of a similar clinical type the child needed Vitamin B 6. We need many non-caloric nutrients in our diet that make up the total "spark plug" that enables our cells to function properly and efficiently.

Crib death, Sudden Infant Death Syndrome (SIDS), remains a modern mystery. An ostensibly healthy infant is found dead by his parent in the morning. He (it is commoner in boys) died during the night and no obvious clues are visible. Only microscopic changes are found in the brain stem, part of the computer brain. These are considered to be what is called agonal, meaning that they are produced by deficiency of oxygen at the time of death and are not evidence of cause.

For a long time most investigators had not accepted the fact that an infant could demonstrate symptoms that might herald this awful event. On several occasions, I had experienced cases where the parents had heard their infant gasp and noted that he was cyanotic (blue due to lack of oxygen) and not breathing. They would pick him up and perhaps smack his buttock and he would revive and start breathing again. The infant would be rushed to the nearest emergency room where nothing abnormal could be found and the infant would be sent home. On a number of occasions, this history had been repeated in a single infant and the parents would actually take shifts throughout the night to ensure that this would not happen while they were themselves asleep.

An article in the prestigious *British Medical Journal* was written in the 1940s by a British public health physician who had investigated sudden death in the breast fed infants of Chinese mothers in Hong Kong. The epidemiology was identical to that reported constantly in modern SIDS. In the Chinese babies it was shown to be infantile beriberi due to lack of Vitamin B1 in breast milk. Because of this discovery, I started to give infants with this kind of history fairly large doses of Vitamin B1 and found that their symptoms cleared up.

Dr. David Read, a physiologist in the University of Sidney had discovered much the same thing and was interested in the role of Vitamin B1 causing SIDS. In attempting to find a solution, he had been working with another physician who was in charge of the laboratory in Australia that does all the blood vitamin assays. Dr. Read had sent him blood samples from some of the SIDS infants that he had encountered and a strange thing was found. These infants almost always had extremely elevated concentrations of Vitamin B1 in their blood, a phenomenon that obviously tended to refute the idea that this vitamin was lacking.

A New Zealand pediatrician had found SIDS to be rather common in his practice area. He collected blood samples from twenty infants dying of a multitude of different conditions. He coded them all with numbers and sent them to the Australian laboratory to have the Vitamin B1 measured. Within the group this physician knew that there were three SIDS infants and the laboratory had no idea what was the cause of death in any. Two of them could easily be picked out because the Vitamin B1 level was so high that the contrast with all the other samples was quite irrefutable.

Since Vitamin B1 given to infants had stopped their symptoms, this was an anachronism and the explanation may depend on an understanding of the metabolism of Vitamin B1. Thiamin is its biochemical name and it has to have the addition of molecules of phosphate in order to become active as a vitamin. We concluded that it was the absence of this action, known as *phosphorylation*, that had resulted in the vitamin being biologically inactive, the equivalent of thiamin deficiency. If a vitamin is not activated and made available to the cellular machinery, it can collect in the system. It could then be in high concentration in the blood, but not doing the work that is required to create energy. It appears to be similar to the collection of folic acid and B12 in the blood of the child described above. They were there but not being used effectively. By giving large doses of Vitamin B1, perhaps some of the vitamin was being processed and activated but in insufficient quantity. By increasing the amount of vitamin given to the infant, perhaps the processing was then sufficient to activate it.

Since then, there have been several papers that suggest other biochemical mechanisms in SIDS, all of which are integral in the biochemistry of energy metabolism. I strongly suspect that these babies die because the Vitamin B1 is there, but unusable because some other missing nutrient factor is required. This could be magnesium since the vitamin is heavily dependent upon its association with this mineral. It is not surprising, therefore, that Dr. Joan Cadell wrote several papers on magnesium deficiency as the cause of SIDS. Her work, which was produced in a scholarly and professional way, was ignored and the problem of SIDS is still considered a mystery. This is largely because mainstream medicine has resolutely refused to believe all the evidence that has accumulated on the therapeutic importance of nutrition. Without the catalysts that enable oxygen to be consumed, the microscopic evidence in the brain stem of these infants is, in my view, evidence of inefficient oxidation, not insufficient oxygen. Yes, it is true that positioning the infant in the crib has cut down the incidence of SIDS but there is still a recognizable incidence of this tragedy, the majority of which occur in the low socioeconomic families where the best nutrition is beyond their means. Giving a few simple vitamin nutrients to an infant that has excessive irritability, a warning sign of his potential for SIDS, seems to be a pediatrician's obvious action since there is no harm involved, even if the irritability is a false sign of risk.

A fifteen-year old boy had loss of appetite, fatigue, abdominal pain, and weight loss. Taking any food at all caused him to have nausea. Because of extreme fatigue he would go to bed early, often without having anything to eat. He had a constantly congested nose, spasms of coughing, recurrent hoarseness, was nervous and irritable. He was constantly "cracking his knuckles," a habit that is often irritatingly repetitive in adolescents. He suffered from headaches, abdominal pain, and nausea to the point of vomiting, particularly with exercise as in running track. About half way around an athletic track he would pull off, vomit, and then continue running. He began to miss school and had been admitted to a hospital for study. The family had been told that a blood test showed liver damage.

His diet was the major clue, but nobody had ever bothered to take a diet history. He subsisted on cookies, potato chips, consumed two gallons of milk and one gallon of carbonated sodas a week. I was able to hear his pulse with my stethoscope applied to his groin (the femoral pulse) and his blood pressure was 130/20, yielding a pulse pressure of 110 (the difference between the two pressures). After dietary instruction and a few vitamin supplements his blood pressure became 120/60 one month later and nausea, abdominal pain and headache had disappeared. It is necessary to point out that the pulse pressure had fallen by fifty points.

It was quite clear that this was a severely disordered limbic system computer, thus explaining the irritability, headache, nausea, vomiting, and even the compulsive knuckle cracking. The blood pressure had been changed by an abnormal balance in the autonomic nervous system. Beriberi, the nutritional disease that upsets the balance of the autonomic nervous system, is an example of high calorie carbohydrate malnutrition. Thiamin is necessary in the processing of glucose in the body and the excess of carbohydrate overwhelms the mechanisms involved, thus inducing relative thiamin deficiency. This boy's high calorie malnutrition was similar to the early stages of beriberi, one of the major causes of so much irritable and incomprehensible behavior in so many people, particularly children and adolescents.

The nutritional diseases like beriberi have been considered to have been abolished, making it impossible for the modern American physician to consider it as a diagnostic possibility.

The consensus is that the last place on earth where malnutrition can be found is in middle class America. One of the tests that I performed on this boy was a glucose tolerance, a test that is familiar to many. It is often used in the detection of diabetes. The blood is tested for its sugar content while fasting and the patient is then given sugar and the blood test repeated at the half hour and again at one, two, three, four and sometimes five hours. Under normal conditions, the blood sugar will increase after the sugar is ingested, rising to a peak at about one hour. It should then gradually decrease and be more or less back to the fasting level at about two hours and thereafter. In this boy, the blood sugar levels remained much the same throughout the test period, giving a "flat" glucose tolerance result.

I repeated the tolerance but took the blood sugar level every ten minutes throughout the first hour. It rose sharply to its peak at about twenty minutes and was back to the fasting level at the half-hour.

The mechanism is easy to understand. When we take sugar, the limbic computer senses the change. It then sends a signal to the gland cells that produce insulin, the hormone that causes sugar to be taken into body cells and used as fuel or stored. In this boy, his diet had made his brain highly reactive to incoming stimuli, including its perception of a rise in sugar content of his blood. Because of this, the message sent out by his brain was exaggerated, resulting in an excess of insulin being produced. This "buried" the sugar in his body cells very quickly and because the first blood drawn after sugar ingestion during the tolerance test is at the half- hour, the peak was missed and the entire test was "flat." In short, this was completely in keeping with the concept that the boy's brain was in a state of irritability to literally any form of stimulus. The irony of it was that it was the consumption of sugar that had caused the situation in the first place.

A Nutritional Approach to a Revised Model for Medicine

As most people know, a person who has the condition of hypoglycemia, a very common problem in today's world, can become faint when hungry and such a person usually requires frequent meals. Because the blood sugar concentration falls steeply at this time and is considered to be the cause of the fainting episode, the usual administered antidote is, of course, sugar. Although this undoubtedly works, it is not the right treatment. It is the ingestion of sugar over a long period of time that has set the computer up to behave abnormally. Sugar works in an emergency situation, but the victim should be informed that ceasing the intake of sugar as a dietary addiction is necessary to stop this kind of event from happening at all. Even in the emergency situation, whole food would work, although its effect would be slower.

In order to understand this apparent paradox, it is necessary to point out that if a person addicted to a street drug, cocaine for example, has withdrawal symptoms, a shot of cocaine will immediately cause those symptoms to cease. This, after all, is the whole principle behind addiction. The more one gets of the addictive drug, the more one needs to prevent the symptoms of withdrawal. Thus, sugar taken in the way that so many people ingest it, becomes a drug. The reason why this has not been taken seriously and is frankly unbelievable to many is because it is the nature of the individual person that matters. It is that person's body chemistry that is more easily affected in some than in others and sugar simply does not have this effect on everyone. This applies to all the addictive drugs. We all know that some people can drink large amounts of alcohol and not become an alcoholic, and it is just as easy for some to stop taking coffee or sugar. Others have a very difficult time in doing this and it is clear that they are addicted. They have withdrawal symptoms if they cease taking the drug. Some people are known to take an occasional shot of cocaine and do not become addicted to it. Naturally, this is a dangerous procedure, but it illustrates the variability of body chemistry from person to person.

Another way of describing this boy is to say that he was maladapted to the environment because his brain computer was not able to "read" the incoming data from his senses properly. It must be emphasized that the brain, not the stomach, caused his attacks of vomiting when running track. I have seen young people who feel hot when they should feel cold and vice versa. The principle can be extended to an explanation for so many of the conditions that are usually termed neurosis. High calorie malnutrition is like having a permanently choked engine in a car. The ability to burn fuel is compromised and the main impact is made upon the "oxygen hungry" tissues of the brain, particularly the lower computer brain.

Perhaps the most startling example of high calorie malnutrition that I have ever witnessed was in an anesthesiologist in his sixties. He had been assessed in his own hospital because of heart failure and subjected to heart catheterization to ascertain whether he had coronary obstruction. To the surprise of the cardiologists, his arterial system was in excellent condition and the cause was not determined. His son was in medical school and he took his father's history to the library to research it. He then announced that the condition that afflicted him was beriberi, the ancient scourge of rice consuming cultures. This produced profound skepticism, but for the first time someone had looked seriously at the diet of this physician and an extraordinary story unfolded. He would get up in the morning and, because of nausea, he would have no breakfast. When he went to the garage to get into his car, he would have "the dry heaves," vomiting with an empty stomach. On arrival at the hospital, he would proceed to the operating room where he would perform anesthesia for perhaps ten or eleven cases. At about four p.m., after the surgical list was ended, he would go to a snack bar and eat a large piece of chocolate cake. When he got home in the evening, he would be so tired that he could not be bothered to eat, or else he would cut some slices of beef (he owned a beef cattle ranch) and go to bed exhausted.

A Nutritional Approach to a Revised Model for Medicine

Giving the correct vitamins to someone as ill as this could be an extremely tricky business. As the metabolism begins to increase, the worn out organs, including the heart, have difficulty in responding. This might be compared with a person who knows that he has an abnormal noise in the engine of his car and drives it to a service station rapidly. Obviously, he risks having more serious damage to the engine. His physicians were eventually persuaded that his son's diagnosis was correct. Although vitamins were administered, no proper precautions were taken to safeguard this difficult period of treatment, and he died from cardiac arrest.

In order to understand the extraordinary resistance and profound ignorance of doctors in the realm of this kind of life-threatening malnutrition, the physician's death was seen as an effect of giving him the vitamins. Unfortunately, that was absolutely correct. The dangerous period is when the brain/body function begins to awaken and the adaptive signals go out to the body from the brain computer. Since that time, I have learned that vitamin treatment will give rise to this kind of difficult period for many people on initiation. When I treat someone nutritionally for asthma, for example, I always warn the patient that things may become worse before they get better. During the first month or so of treatment, there may be an acute attack of asthma, requiring a visit to the emergency room. Like the formula proposed by Buddhists, "you have to go though Hell to get to Nirvana." In more modern terms, I have given this reaction the term "paradox" because it is the opposite of what is expected.

The orthodox medical model states that the physician who is "controlling" the disease knows what he is doing. Therefore, if a patient has an adverse reaction at the beginning of treatment, he is going to assume that the doctor does not know what he is doing! It is tacitly assumed that this is a "side reaction" to the vitamins, which are often referred to as "the medication." It creates a difficulty in the physician/patient trust relationship that is obvious. Today, I always warn my patients that they may have some recurrence of their symptoms at the outset of treatment and this is the only period of vitamin administration that needs to be "managed."

Here is another example of a nutritional approach. A seven-year old boy had been hyperactive since the age of ten months. Night terrors and sleep walking were common while sleep walking was accompanied by profuse sweating and involuntary urination. Fever had been noted in association with a night terror and occurred sometimes with a migraine-like headache that affected one side of his head. He had a short attention span, although psychological testing revealed a high-grade intelligence quotient. Knee jerks were too brisk, sometimes double in character and often "hung up." This is a very simple test that I use in all children with this kind of affliction, and is used by physicians always in a routine physical examination because it tests important aspects of reflex nervous system activity. The tendon just below the knee-cap is tapped, usually with a rubber headed hammer a familiar event for almost anybody. As a result, a message is conveyed to the reflex nervous system that comes back in a signal to the thigh muscle to contract. The lower leg gives a little kick forwards and the amount of movement is proportional to the power of the nervous impulse that causes it. It is possible to get a judgment on the degree of sensitivity of the nervous mechanisms that control this reflex and in this case, his reflex activity was super-sensitive. In some children the knee jerks twice or even three times. I can only interpret that as a signal that goes back and forth through the reflex apparatus in much the same way as ripples on the surface of a pond will respond when a stone is thrown into the water. As the ripples hit an obstruction or the bank of the pond, they are reflected back. *Hyper-reflexia*, literally meaning "too much reflex" as this is called, is not a normal phenomenon and indicates irritability or increased sensitivity of the system.

I mentioned here that the reflex was occasionally "hung up" and this is also abnormal, a feature also seen in the disease known as St. Vitus Dance, or Chorea as the medical books call it. As the knee tendon is tapped, the leg kicks forwards but the muscle does not relax and the leg remains "hung up" for a while before it drops back into its original position. This is most easily seen when the examiner puts one arm under the thigh and holds it up while eliciting the reflex with the other hand. In some children, I have seen the reflex take place without actually tapping the tendon. This is done by stopping the hammer short of actually making contact. In fact, it can only be assumed that the reflex takes place because the child sees the action and his brain "expects" it. This must mean that the action can be initiated through a visual signal and implies that the brain is involved in that action.

The value of this in assessing the problem in a hyperactive child is because it is pointing clearly to the fact that the nervous system is disordered. The behavior of such a child, which is so frequently assumed to be "annoying" and perpetrated voluntarily, is brought about by a compulsion that is a feature of lower brain activity and is not willed. It has nothing to do with classical psychology and talk therapy. Punishment and traditional methods of treatment have little or no bearing on it. In fact, punishment usually ends up by making things much worse as the child becomes more and more frustrated by what he correctly perceives as misunderstanding of his plight. The attempts to punish him only increase the stress as we have already defined that word.

I have already indicated that the blood pressure can be a valuable tool. In a previous chapter, we discussed the difference between blood pressure and pulse pressure, the latter being the most important aspect of an examination in so many of these children. In this child, the blood pressure was 114/20 (measured as always by millimeters of mercury) and it will be remembered that the pulse pressure is derived by subtracting the lower figure from the upper one. So this pressure was ninety-four in this child, much too high.

The child was heavily indulged with sweets and soft drinks. Diabetes was present on both sides of the family and I have found this family history often to be a pointer to sugar sensitivity within family members. After rescheduling his diet and making sure that all the "junk" was removed, together with a few supplementary vitamins that included Vitamin B1, his symptoms cleared completely, and his blood pressure returned to a comfortable 90/60 (pulse pressure thirty).

This case must be discussed in light of the model that I have proposed. Many will remember that they were told early on in childhood that night terrors were caused by certain foods taken in the evening before bedtime. What I have observed is that there is not usually a direct cause and effect relationship between taking a specific food in this manner. But certain foods, the worst being the sweets, set the limbic brain up in the way that has already been discussed, so that it is much more reactive to incoming stimuli. A night terror is certainly governed from this part of the brain and, again, it has nothing to do with psychology. It is a bad dream associated with physical accompaniment actuated through the autonomic nervous system. A child might sit up in bed, crying, or screaming. He will appear to be wide-awake and the pupils dilated. He might be sweating profusely and his heart racing. It is a typical "fight-or-flight" reflex actuated in the computer spontaneously during sleep. It will be remembered that this reflex is an important one when there is real danger. In the case of a night terror it is the abnormal sensitivity of the computer that fires the reflex without any actual threat.

The pulse pressure is a pure function of this part of the brain as well, and is evidence that the reflex mechanisms that occur between the heart, the brain, and the nervous control of blood vessel contraction/dilatation are at variance and poorly coordinated. In short, such a child is poorly adapted to his environment and is easily made sick, physically, mentally or both. Mental is physical and physical is mental because they are inextricably locked together in regulating all functions of the body. It should also be noted that the child urinating involuntarily while sleep walking was because of a "trigger happy" nervous system regulated by the limbic brain. I have seen this a number of times and it is very much the same kind of reflex pattern that causes bed-wetting or enuresis, something that occurs during sleep.

How can he be unconscious while walking downstairs? A great deal of human activity is controlled from the lower brain and the conscious or cognitive brain can be merely a "helpless observer" if the person is conscious, and totally unaware if unconscious. By that, I mean that some activities are often seen as volitional, whereas they are actually driven by the primitive brain. The sophisticated brain might be inactive as in the perpetration of induced anger leading to murder, or it might be fully aware of the action, but powerless to stop it. We can then refer to the action as "a compulsion." If the cognitive brain is impaired enough, there may be no evidence of remorse from the person performing an act of violence.

The migraine headaches ceased in the case of the child just described. This type of headache is caused by a lack of balance in the autonomic system that controls the caliber of the small blood vessels that supply the scalp. There is an additional reaction that takes place in the blood vessels that causes the liquid part of the blood to leak out into the tissues and cause local swelling, or *edema*. In some cases, this edema can easily be found by pressing a finger into the painful area and maintaining that pressure for a little while, thus increasing the pain. After the pressure is released, a small dimple can be found where the finger was applied, thus indicating that the tissue was swollen with edema. This edema is caused from the release of pro-inflammatory prostaglandins acting on the blood vessels and that mechanism causes pain.

One last comment that can be extracted from the case of this child is that his intelligence quotient (I.Q.) was high. Most of the children with conditions of this nature are intelligent, but their academic, and sometimes their athletic potential is impaired. The reason is really quite simple. I repeat that you cannot put poor fuel into a well-made machine. The human brain uses massive amounts of oxygen in order to carry out its continuous function and it is a measure of its high metabolic rate. That is why mental fatigue is even more tiring than physical fatigue and it also feels different. Most people know that sitting at a desk and doing mental work is much more fatiguing than physical work. The limbic brain becomes irritable if it is de-energized and it is the secret of understanding the epidemic of brain syndromes that are seen in our children today. The easiest way to de-energize is through the consumption of "junk" food and beverages.

One of the major difficulties that I have in giving explanations to patients is the fact that "mental" is just as "physical" as "physical" is "mental." This is because literally nothing happens in the body without the brain being involved. If so-called mental symptoms appear to be the dominating feature, the patient is traditionally regarded as a psychiatric case and either talk therapy or drug treatment is offered. This prevailing attitude makes it almost impossible for society to accept crime, committed in anger, as an illness of the mind. It also interferes with our perception of the effects of a whiplash injury, for example.

I have seen a number of people who have had prolonged symptoms following a whiplash. They complain of fatigue, pain, and stiffness in the neck and shoulder muscles, and they simply do not return to the state of health that they were in before the injury.

Since litigation or an insurance claim is almost always involved, the general attitude toward such people is that they are "trying to extract as much money from the offending party as possible." This automatically introduces the suspicion of malingering, though this is never said openly. It is merely inferred by the long road of legal posturing that follows a person attempting to obtain proper redress that the victim associates with the accident.

A Nutritional Approach to a Revised Model for Medicine

The evidence that I have accumulated is that this perception by society, as it exists at present, is in most cases quite erroneous. When the brain is involved in a shake-up of this nature, its computer control is severely affected. It results in unusual and unnecessary messages being flashed out and they result in body organ activity that becomes interpreted as a "psychosomatic" condition. Obeying the teaching of traditional psychology, this is then seen as what is known as secondary gain. The patient is considered to be using symptoms to prolong the after effects "to gain attention." The patients that I have seen in this situation are almost invariably weary of being considered in this framework. Nothing that they say or do deflects the prevailing opinion of both their legal and medical advisors. Traditional studies are done repeatedly, such as CAT scans, MRIs, X-rays, and blood tests. Because all are normal, it is deduced that nothing is wrong and the symptoms must be generated "psychologically." No matter where they go or whom they consult, they are labeled in this way and there appears to be no escape.

Unfortunately, this is the fate so many people have when they suffer from the somewhat tenuous diagnostic categories of Chemical Sensitivity Syndrome, Chronic Fatigue Syndrome, and Fibromyalgia Syndrome. All of these are merely "variations on a symphonic theme," that theme being an energy crisis which is often induced iatrogenically (physician produced) by the unwise and persistent use of powerful antibiotics that were probably not needed in the first place. The reader is urged to go back to the chapter that dealt with energy metabolism and review the topic of mitochondria.

The worst example of this was in the parents of two children who had a genetically determined disease that causes mental retardation. The parents were both carriers of the recessive gene that, when given to the child in a double dose (one gene from each parent), would result in the appearance of the disease. It so happens that this condition affects the brain stem computer and is partially responsive to high doses of vitamins, particularly B1.

Derrick Lonsdale M.D.

The prevailing opinion is that a carrier state is totally free of risk because "the one good gene that the person has will take care of the activity of the missing one." It is true that if someone loses a lung, the other one will compensate, but the affected person would not be expected to be a good athlete, for example. This particular disease is quite rare and is difficult to recognize, like most of the genetically determined disease

Inborn Errors of Metabolism

This couple had two severely retarded children with one abnormal gene from each parent, but because they were "carriers" they appeared to be clinically normal. The prevailing opinion is that any illness or event in their lives would not be considered related in any way to their carrier state. The father, who was in his late thirties at the time, was hit by a car and was thrown some distance. No bones were broken and it was considered to be a "lucky escape" from death or serious injury. After this, he had extreme stiffness and muscular pain in many muscles, particularly in the neck and shoulder region. He sought relief from many quarters and was treated with physical therapy, massage, and other such techniques, to no avail. One day, as he was desperately attempting his own rehabilitation, he entered a racket ball court by himself for exercise. He was subsequently found dead in a toilet. Autopsy revealed that there was some *aortic stenosis* (a narrowing of the main blood vessel from the heart) and this is known to be associated with sudden death, although the reason is quite unclear.

Although his life insurance carried double accident indemnity, it was ruled that the severe accident that he had sustained some months previously was not a factor and that double indemnity did not apply. I notified the insurance company that his death would not have occurred if he had not been in an accident, that this was an extreme form of stress which had affected his energy metabolism.

Fibromyalgia is known to be caused by defective mitochondrial activity. This example again shows us how the Three Circles of Health operate together.

His widow was a flight attendant and she carried on her career with success for some years, but then began to show rapidly developing signs of premature aging. She suffered from extreme fatigue, made worse by flying. Nutritional therapy helped her to regain her health after she was grounded, although the airline that employed her refused to recognize this for a long time. Being a carrier of the gene was not enough to cause the classic expression of the full-blown disease but the increased energy demand of stress was impaired. In the case of the father, the accident became the stressor on top of his genetic risk, while in the mother, flying in the diminished oxygen concentration and re-circulated air, were responsible.

Energy metabolism is the real key to understanding so many things in medicine that we presently ignore. We live in a perpetually hostile environment to which we have to adapt continuously, twenty-four hours a day. Each adaptive strategy is coordinated and put into action by the computer in the brain, a "machine" that requires an inordinate amount of oxygen and nutrients. The greater the stress, the greater the required defensive response and hence the more energy that is consumed. This is no different from a car that has to climb a hill. It has to work harder, consume more fuel, and produce more heat in the effort. If the engine is impaired for any reason, its task is more difficult and it may develop symptoms that are easily recognized by the driver. Symptoms in the human organism can be analogically compared with those of the car. They are evidence of a struggle to "make energy ends meet."

My two patients, described above, represent casualties of present ignorance that should not exist. If they are looked at as being born, with a gene "mistake" that contains a hidden weakness in their ability to create energy from fuel, the picture is seen differently. The fact that they each delivered this recessive gene to each of their two children was not their fault, but created a serious energy loss in the brains of the children and resulted in their mental retardation. The "good" gene, which both parents possessed within their genetic constitution, was sufficient to perform the work of two genes, but only under normal, non-stressful living conditions. The overlay of stresses described made the difference. Each, by the present disease model, would be treated as separate and totally unrelated illnesses and the stress relationship disregarded. It can easily be seen why the insurance company would not accept double indemnity for an association with the accident, and why the airline could not see the reason their employee was unable to fly.

Here is another example of the brain/body mechanism. A five-year old boy had recurrent episodes of vomiting. At the age of three, he had complained of aches and pains in the legs and would cry because of them. Swelling of the feet and ankles had prevented him from wearing shoes and the appearance of a rash led to a diagnosis of "rheumatic fever." He had received injections of penicillin for six months, although an active streptococcal infection, always an associated factor in this disease, was never proved and he continued to complain of the pains. He would awaken in the morning feeling unwell and ask for a drink that he would promptly vomit. Recurrent vomiting would continue for the subsequent twelve hours with a high body temperature. Occasionally he would become rigid and stiff for a few minutes. Touching him made him scream on these occasions and the entire event would end with him "being exhausted." Night terrors and talking about violence occurred in sleep and on one occasion he cried out that he was unable to move because he felt that he was pinned down by a wild animal. At other times his legs repeatedly jerked when he was asleep. A rapid heart beat had been noted with the vomiting attacks and his appetite was capricious and unpredictable. After the administration of Vitamin B1 and supervision of his diet, the symptoms all disappeared.

A Nutritional Approach to a Revised Model for Medicine

This kind of repetitive vomiting, known as cyclic vomiting, occurs in children and it is known to be associated with functional changes in activity of the autonomic nervous system. All his symptoms were understandable if perceived as arising from the computer. The rapid heart-beat was generated by a reaction in the sympathetic branch of the autonomic nervous system. The irritable leg in sleep, referred to as "jumping leg syndrome" is a common problem. This, the night terrors and the vomiting were all caused by a biochemical disturbance in that part of the brain.

Perhaps the most interesting symptom was that of his perception of "being pinned down by a wild animal." The human brain goes through some very complex electro-chemical reactions when we are asleep and a night's sleep is divided up into a number of phases called sleep cycles. A complete cycle lasts about ninety minutes, and it is divided into two separate sections, known as rapid eye movement sleep (REM) which lasts about ten minutes, and non-REM sleep which takes up the other eighty minutes. The non-REM component is known as deep sleep and it goes through several stages of depth. The fascinating part of the cycle is REM, even though it is only ten minutes out of the total. It is this phase, also known as "active sleep," which appears to be the most important for health. It may be a vital part of building energy stores, if a person is deprived of REM activity repeatedly for a long enough time, he will die.

During REM sleep puzzling physiological things take place. The autonomic system becomes extremely active, generating functional changes in the body. It is only in this phase that we dream. Abnormal biochemistry and physiology of the part of the brain from which this is controlled causes a number of disorders. One of these is known as sleep paralysis. An affected person awakens while in the REM sleep state, unable to move any part of the body consciously for a time. Recovery occurs spontaneously. In the case of the child, it may have been a dream that gave him the explanation of feeling pinned down. It would obviously be very frightening to him. The point is that all of the symptoms that this child suffered were because of a biochemically deranged brain. The cause could easily be removed by introducing a normal diet and providing a vitamin that plays an essential part in governing energy metabolism, particularly in the automatic brain that must continue to govern our bodily functions while we are asleep.

Another of these conditions is called *sleep apnea*. The sufferer stops breathing (apnea), something that might not be noticed at all by the patient, who remains asleep. Breathing ceases for as long as ten to fifteen seconds, followed by a sudden deep breath, perhaps accompanied by a snore, gasping or suddenly sitting up in bed, even though still asleep. It is caused by the brain computer becoming less sensitive to carbon dioxide. Breathing stops because the carbon dioxide drive is insufficient to maintain the mechanism. After breathing stops, carbon dioxide builds up in the blood circulating through the computer. As it finally reaches a concentration that is sufficient to stimulate the brain mechanism into activity, a "panic" message goes out from the computer, and the patient takes a sudden deep breath. He may awaken at this time, starting out of sleep, and sitting up in bed.

Sleep apnea was discovered because a woman complained that evil spirits were attacking her husband while he was asleep. He would suddenly sit up in bed, clutching this throat with a huge gasp, then drop back onto the bed, and continue to snore loudly as many people with this affliction do. He was finally investigated in a sleep laboratory when the mechanism became clear. I have seen a number of these patients and have witnessed their complete recovery after correcting their diet and supplying them with appropriate vitamin/mineral supplements. It is another example of inefficient metabolism in a part of the brain that is critical to life itself. Because of the biochemical derangement that occurs in the wake of years of high calorie malnutrition, the automatic mechanisms that maintain our breathing when unconscious during sleep fail. In some cases there undoubtedly is genetic predisposition, making them prone to its clinical

A Nutritional Approach to a Revised Model for Medicine

expression because of bad diet and lifestyle, another example of the Three Circles of Health.

Some children awaken at night screaming with pain in the legs or knees. The mother goes to the child's room where she soothes him by massaging the leg. Such pains used to be called growing pains, but that explanation fell out of favor, though the cause was never better elucidated. This kind of pain is indeed associated with rapid growth, insufficiently supported by adequate nutritional intake. This was most vividly brought home to me when I saw a child who would literally scream from such pain in the middle of the night. He also had learning disability that had resulted in his mother schooling him at home. The paradox was that he had an extremely high IQ and was brilliant enough that he had gone to the library at the age of five and written an essay on birds of prey. It was another example of the nutritional requirements of a well developed brilliant brain and he did well when the diet was improved and supplementary nutrients supplied.

We only know the world in which we live because of electrochemical reactions in the brain that have to be interpreted. Vision, hearing, sensing smells, and tactile stimulation all depend on complex nerve pathways to the brain where the signals are decoded and interpreted. So does the world around us really exist? We only know that it is there because of an interpretation by our brains, a very old philosophical riddle. Since those perceptions are totally dependent upon a normal programmed brain reaction, abnormal chemistry will give rise to abnormal perceptions. Do we all "see" the world in the same way? We do not know. We merely assume that it is so. If a person has been programmed to call a given color "red," he will always see that particular perception as the color "red." Does another person see something different and call it red?

I must describe one of the most interesting and frustrating cases in my experience. The patient, when first seen, was six-years of age. He had come through a bad birth situation during which there had been clear evidence of a lack of oxidation. This is usually felt most by the brain and is the reason for many children being born with what is known as cerebral palsy. In this child, hyperactivity, short attention span, an intense sensitivity to sound, and periodic wheezing developed in early childhood. He was considered to be mentally retarded.

At the age of twelve he had been admitted to a hospital with a transient incident that had been called a stroke. (When this occurs in older adults it is called a *Transient Ischemic Attack*, often referred to a "TIA.") This had been preceded by a loss of appetite, lethargy, vomiting, diarrhea, abdominal pain, and heart palpitations. About ten days after discharge from hospital his parents took him on a picnic in mountainous country. While sitting at a picnic table in the heat of the sun, he again developed weakness of the right arm and leg, left facial weakness, and drooling. This recovered quickly while he was being transported to hospital in an air-conditioned car. Note that the hot sun would be a source of physical stress to the child under these circumstances. Studies in the hospital revealed an enlarged heart and the illness then began to imitate the nutritional disease known as beriberi.

He responded initially to large doses of Vitamin B1 given by injection. The enlarged heart reduced to normal size and all his symptoms cleared up with the continuation of very large doses of this vitamin, deficiency of which is known to be associated with beriberi. This was, however, short lived and he began to relapse. He died eventually from a typical imitation of the condition known by the Japanese as *shoshin*. This is a form of extremely acute beriberi, the most lethal form of the disease. This boy did not have a dietary vitamin deficiency. It was a genetically determined dependency on a balance of non-caloric nutrients that could not be determined in the state of knowledge at that time. The point is that his lethal disease exactly imitated the pathophysiology that would be seen in classical beriberi.

A Nutritional Approach to a Revised Model for Medicine

The history of beriberi when it was in epidemic form in China is of some interest. It occurred commonly in hard working laborers in the factories who were subsisting on a diet of white rice. The workers would take their lunch in a corridor between the factory buildings. They would initially be in the shade, but if the sun began to shine down on them some of them would develop the first symptoms of the disease. It was because of the appearance of these first symptoms in a group of people at the same time that made the clinicians of the day think that beriberi was an infection. It was therefore important to note that the illness in the boy just described developed symptoms as he was sitting at a picnic table in the heat of the sun.

Again, we are looking at the Three Circles of Health where sunlight was the stressor that initiated the disease when the underlying body chemistry was marginal. Since the body is a biochemical "machine" it must ultimately be the biochemist who must ignore the symptoms and find the underlying basic cause of all of them. It is no longer sufficient to make a clinical diagnosis in the form that we use today. Some will remember the parable of the "blind men and the elephant." A group of blind men were asked to describe an elephant. One got the ear: another got the trunk and another, the leg or the tail. Each described the part he examined with great accuracy, thinking that he had described the elephant but could not know that he had missed the "big picture." Perhaps we are missing the real "elephant" in present day medicine!

CONCLUSION

High calorie malnutrition may be of extraordinary importance since it could explain some of the things about ourselves that we cannot presently understand. Can it explain some of the inexplicable crimes of passion, for instance? Could it be a powerful factor in the widespread problem of senseless vandalism? That is the reason that I have attempted to compare the decline of Roman Civilization through lead poisoning to the decline in our own through the dangerously destructive mechanisms caused by this form of malnutrition. It is not seen as malnutrition because we are not hungry as in starvation. If anything can be blamed it is our inveterate hedonism, our love of pleasurable sensation. Sugar and all forms of sweeteners send a hedonistic signal into that part of the brain that provides the pleasure and which makes it into a drug when we ingest it in all its different forms. Extracting an active principle from a plant turns it into a drug. Peruvian Indians chew coca leaves that enable them to live and survive at great heights in the Andes. They do not get the illness associated with taking cocaine, the active principle of the leaf. This indicates that the extraction of an active principle from a plant source alters the action of the active principle. The whole plant, taken as an herb, has a different action.

###

www.ingramcontent.com/pod-product-compliance
Lightning Source LLC
LaVergne TN
LVHW040719060525
810504LV00006B/93